The complete guide to
female
FERTILITY

KATE BRIAN

PIATKUS

The opinions and advice expressed in this book are intended as a guide only. Neither the publisher nor the author is engaged in rendering professional advice or services to the individual reader. The publisher and author accept no responsibility for any injury or loss sustained as a result of using this book.

Copyright © 2007 by Kate Brian
First published in 2007 by
Piatkus Books Ltd
5 Windmill Street
London W1T 2JA
Email: info@piatkus.co.uk

The moral right of the author has been asserted
A catalogue record for this book is available from the British Library.

The suggestions and treatments described in this book should not replace the care and direct supervision of a trained healthcare professional. If you have any pre-existing health problem or if you are currently taking medications of any sort, you should consult your doctor or equivalent health professional prior to following the suggestions in this book. The recommendations given in this book are intended solely as education and information, and should not be taken as medical advice. Neither the author nor the publisher accept liability for readers who choose to self-prescribe.

ISBN 978 0 7499 2792 9

Medical advice from Richard Howell, FRCOG, Consultant Gynaecologist, Brighton and Sussex University Hospitals NHS Trust and The Agora Gynaecology and Fertility Centre, Brighton and Hove

Edited by Jan Cutler
Text design by Goldust Design

This book has been printed on paper manufactured with respect for the environment using wood from managed sustainable resources.

Printed and bound in Great Britain by
William Clowes Ltd, Beccles, Suffolk

To Max, Alfie and Flora

Kate Brian is a writer and journalist who specialises in issues surrounding female fertility. She is a member of the board of Infertility Network UK, and has worked with the charity on a number of projects. She has been a member of a Human Fertilisation and Embryology Authority expert advisory group, and a trustee of CHILD (infertility charity). Kate is a former Home Affairs producer for Channel 4 News and now writes features for national newspapers and magazines. She has two children who were born after IVF treatment.

Contents

Acknowledgements

I want to say a huge thank you to all the women who agreed to talk to me for this book. I had so many fascinating conversations with so many lovely women, and was struck again and again by your courage in all kinds of difficult circumstances, and your generosity in sharing your personal experiences. Although not all the interviews appear in the final version of the book, everyone provided new insights and ideas, and I'm very grateful to you all.

I am indebted to Judy Piatkus, Alice Davis and Diana Tyler for making this happen, and to Richard Howell for agreeing to help me once again – not only giving medical advice and suggestions but also spotting my typing errors. Thanks to Clare Brown, Chief Executive of Infertility Network UK, who has been a source of inspiration over many years, and Susan Seenan of Infertility Network UK for her hard work and patience. Thanks also to Rachel Hawkes of Verity, Olivia Montuschi of the Donor Conception Network, to Emily Engel, and to all those who helped me from Single Parent Action Network, netmums.com, mothers35plus.co.uk, asher-mans.org, Single Mothers by Choice, Stonewall, British Association for Adoption and Fostering, Kidding Aside and Young Mums to Be at JHP Training in Nottingham. The expert knowledge of the members of the HFEA multiple births advisory group, Charlotte Augst and Juliet Tizzard, has filtered through into many places in this book, so thanks to you all.

On a personal note, thanks to Graham Binns for spending an evening rescuing my manuscript from the depths of a dying computer, to Jacqui Freeman for spare iMac parts, to Anna McCord, Charles and Sam Meth for escapes to the sun, to Christine Oldfield for her support and to my book club friends (Liz, Kate, Shona, Diana, Sam, Xanthe, Sue, Cheryl, Maureen and Caroline) and Halstow book club friends for giving me an excuse to read something other than medical textbooks. Thank you to my mother Daphne McCord for her help, and most of all my love and thanks as always to Max, and to Alfie and Flora, who have put up with me admirably.

Introduction

Today, we grow up believing that becoming a mother should be just one aspect of a fulfilling life, and it is not something we expect to have to give up everything else to achieve. Many of us choose to delay motherhood until we feel we are ready for it. We may want to make sure we have met the right partner, to establish our careers, travel and enjoy our social lives before settling down to the responsibilities of a family of our own.

I'd always known I wanted to have children one day, but it wasn't until I hit 30 that I was suddenly overwhelmed by the certainty that this was the moment to start trying for a baby. The time had never seemed right before. My partner and I had both been busy with our jobs, and making an active decision to have children seemed a huge commitment, but finally we were ready, and looking forward to becoming parents.

When just a few months had passed and nothing had happened, I decided to take the matter in hand. I specialised in health in my job as a television journalist, and was aware that there were often long waiting lists for fertility treatment, so I began to look into the subject. Soon, we had been referred to our local hospital and we were anticipating some kind of speedy resolution to our situation. Instead, we were faced with one inconclusive test after another, and none of them seemed to get us any closer to finding out why we couldn't have a baby. It was only then that I realised this wasn't going to be as straightforward as I'd anticipated, and that however much research I did, or money we spent, there were no guarantees that we would ever be able to have a child of our own.

After four years of unexplained infertility, six months on clomifene citrate, two IVF attempts and a frozen embryo transfer, I had a positive pregnancy test and went on to give birth to my son. Having a baby was the best thing that had ever happened to me, but getting there had been a lonely, miserable experience and I wanted to do something positive to help others in the same situation. I wrote a book about patient experiences of IVF, *In Pursuit of Parenthood*, as there was no information of this kind available at the time. It led to many requests to give a patient perspective on infertility and treatment, and I learnt more and more about the subject as I spoke to experts in the field, and to others who had personal experience of fertility problems.

When we decided we'd like to see if we could have a second baby, I gave up my job in television and started working freelance. At the same time, I became a trustee of the infertility charity, CHILD, which has since merged with another support group to become Infertility Network UK. We had one more full IVF cycle and four frozen embryo transfers before we were successful again with our daughter.

I found myself becoming ever more fascinated by the whole area of female fertility and the way fertility problems impact on our lives. I worked with Infertility Network UK on a number of projects, writing information leaflets and packs, on patient surveys, media campaigns and training. I wrote articles about infertility for national newspapers and magazines, and was asked to join an expert advisory group which was looking into multiple births after fertility treatment for the Human Fertilisation and Embryology Authority.

I wanted to write this book to help answer the questions women may have about their own fertility. Many of us wonder how late we can leave it to have a baby, whether we are ready to be a mother, and may fear that we will have difficulty conceiving. The book aims to explain the facts and explore some of the dilemmas women face, giving insights into the issues we need to take into account when we are considering starting a family, while also offering practical advice. It looks at how you can boost your chances of getting pregnant, explores what can go wrong and how modern medicine can help. It includes the views of many women who have a wide variety of experiences, and can give insights into different situations and circumstances, from choosing to have a child alone to going through assisted conception. I hope that this book offers something of interest to every woman who wants to know more about her own fertility.

Chapter one

Fertility Basics

Most of us are pretty certain we know the basics already. Our understanding about how women get pregnant probably began with playground gossip and school biology books, perhaps including an embarrassing sit-down chat with our parents along the way, but by the time we reach adulthood we don't need anyone to tell us anything about how babies are made. It's often not until we decide to try it for ourselves that we may realise there are some fairly large gaps in our knowledge about how our reproductive systems work. Do you know how to tell when you're ovulating? Or exactly how many days there are in your cycle when you could get pregnant? Will the method of contraception you've been using make a difference to how quickly you conceive? And how long should it take before you get a positive pregnancy test?

The female reproductive system is complex, and getting pregnant involves a linked chain of events in a woman's body, which begin long before the act of sexual intercourse. A minor imbalance anywhere along the line can cause major problems, and when you look more closely at what has to happen to make a baby, it starts to seem quite incredible that so many women manage to get pregnant without any problems.

Basic terms

It may be helpful to start by looking at the different parts of the female reproductive system, and the role they play in our fertility.

Eggs and ovaries

The word ovary comes from the Latin *ovum*, or egg, and we store our lifetime's supply of eggs in our ovaries. Women have two ovaries, one on either side of their womb, situated just behind it. Each ovary is about the size of a walnut, and the eggs inside are so tiny that they are invisible to the human eye.

Women begin making eggs before they are born. The process starts in the mother's womb when a female embryo is still smaller than a grain of rice, less than a month after fertilisation. By the time a baby girl has been in her mother's womb for five months, her ovaries contain several million eggs, the most they will ever hold. From this point onwards, eggs begin to perish, and by the time a girl is born about half the eggs in her ovaries will have died. This process will carry on throughout her life, and at puberty a girl has half a million eggs at most left in her ovaries. Of these, only four or five hundred will ever mature and have the potential to be fertilised, and the average woman will see fewer than three of them grow into children during her lifetime.

A female's ovaries cannot produce any more eggs once she is born. This means that unlike men, who carry on producing fresh sperm into old age, women are governed by their biological clocks. Towards the end of her reproductive life, a woman is releasing eggs that have been in her body for more than 40 years. She becomes less and less fertile until eventually she stops ovulating (releasing ripe eggs) altogether, sometime between her mid forties and late fifties.

The womb

The uterus, or womb, is the size and shape of an upside-down pear with thick, muscular walls. It is here that a fertilised egg will implant itself and grow, and the womb can stretch to accommodate a growing baby. The womb grows a special soft, spongy lining every month to create the right environment for a fertilised egg to implant, and if this doesn't happen the lining is shed in your period.

The fallopian tubes

Leading from each ovary into the womb are two tiny paths called the fallopian tubes. They are around 10cm (4in) long, and about the thickness of a pin. The end of the tube closest to the ovary has a fluted, funnel shape and is edged with fimbria – delicate fingers that gather up the egg and send it on the journey down the tube. The tube is lined with tiny hair-like cilia that help the egg move towards the womb.

The hypothalamus and pituitary gland

The hypothalamus is a gland in the centre of the brain, and the pituitary gland is situated beneath it at the base of the brain. Together the hypothalamus and pituitary glands orchestrate the production of the hormones that tell the woman's reproductive organs what to do and when to do it.

Puberty

In females, puberty usually begins between the ages of eight and 13. As a girl changes into a woman, her hips widen and her breasts swell, as fat accumulates and milk ducts form inside them. It is 18 months to two years after the start of these signs of puberty that a girl reaches the menarche, when her pituitary gland starts sending out hormones and the menstrual cycle begins.

Periods are often irregular for the first year or two after puberty, because girls don't always start releasing mature eggs immediately. It can take a couple of years before regular ovulation and a fixed menstrual pattern are established.

The menstrual cycle

The word menstruation comes from the Latin *mensis*, or month, and the menstrual cycle (the system of maturing and releasing eggs) is generally considered to be a 28-day process. In fact, each woman has her own individual rhythm and may have a cycle of anything between 25 and 35 days. Some women have even longer or shorter cycles, and many have irregular periods, which can indicate that they are not ovulating normally. The menstrual cycle is regulated by messages sent from the brain. They tell your body when to create the hormones to trigger each stage of the cycle.

The period

The monthly cycle begins when your period starts. The days of the cycle are numbered from the first day of bleeding, so this is known as day one. Your body prepares a soft lining, or endometrium, for your womb every month, just in case you get pregnant. If there is no fertilised egg attached to the womb lining, the levels of progesterone in your body start to fall, and the blood vessels in the endometrium contract. This causes the lining to break up, and it is shed through the neck of the womb, or cervix, into the vagina.

A period may last up to a week, although between three and five days is more usual. It is common to experience some pain or cramping during your period, caused by contractions in the muscles of the womb. One in five women suffer with very heavy bleeding, or menorrhagia, which is defined as a period that lasts more than seven days or during which more than 80 millilitres (2½ fluid ounces) of blood is lost. Most of us have absolutely no idea how many millilitres of blood we lose, or whether our periods are light or heavy compared to other women's. There are wide variations in what is described as 'average' blood loss during a period, but it seems to be anything between a few spoonfuls and half a cup.

During your period, the hypothalamus gland in the brain

starts to release a hormone (the gonadotrophin-releasing hormone or GnRH, for anyone who likes to know the names of these things). This signals the pituitary gland to send out follicle-stimulating hormone, or FSH, which makes the eggs in the ovaries start to grow.

Leading up to ovulation – follicular phase

Initially, as many as 20 eggs may respond to the FSH. Each egg is contained in a little fluid-filled sac, called a follicle. As the follicles start to grow, they send out another hormone: oestrogen. One follicle becomes dominant by about day seven of the cycle, growing faster than the others and releasing more oestrogen. Once the oestrogen reaches a certain level, this alerts the pituitary gland to stop producing so much FSH. The other follicles will then shrink and the eggs inside them die, leaving just the dominant follicle to continue growing. Meanwhile, the lining of the womb, or endometrium, is thickening so that it will be ready in case there is a fertilised embryo to implant.

Ovulation

Once oestrogen levels have reached their highest point, it is time for an egg to be released. It normally takes 14 days from the start of the period to ovulation, but it can take longer for the egg to mature. When the egg is ready, the pituitary gland sends out huge amounts of luteinising hormone, or LH, in a surge that will last 24 hours. The follicle ruptures and the egg is released. Some women know when they ovulate, as they have what is known as Mittelschmerz, or mid-cycle pain. It is usually felt in the lower abdomen, often just inside the hip bone.

The newly released egg is swept up by the fimbria and gathered into the funnel at the end of the fallopian tube, and then begins to travel towards the womb. An egg can survive for only 24 hours once it has been released, so it needs to be fertilised quickly.

Fertilisation

During sexual intercourse as many as 300 million sperm will be ejaculated, but just a tiny percentage – around two hundred at the most – will make it as far as the fallopian tube. The vast majority do not even manage to get through the cervix into the womb.

Once they are inside the female body, sperm can survive for up to a week, although most will not live longer than a couple of days. An egg is more likely to be fertilised if there are fresh sperm ready to meet it in the fallopian tube when it is released.

In order to be able to fertilise an egg, the sperm goes through a process called capacitation. The outer coating of each sperm's head is stripped off, and at the same time the tail stops beating gently and begins to make wide, whiplash beats. This will help the sperm to make its way through the thick outer layer that surrounds the egg. Only the strongest will be able to do this. Once a sperm has successfully got past the outer layers, it binds itself to the egg. Enzymes immediately act on the shell to prevent any other sperm breaking through.

The luteal phase

When an egg has been released, the follicle surrounding it

collapses. Soon it is filled with small cells that proliferate to occupy the space. These cells have a yellow pigment and the mass of cells is called the corpus luteum, or yellow body. The corpus luteum produces progesterone, which helps to build up a thick, healthy womb lining ready for implantation.

Meanwhile, the egg travels down the fallopian tube towards the womb, a journey that takes about a week. If the egg has met a sperm in the tube and been fertilised, it then embeds itself into the womb lining and begins to develop.

If the egg is not fertilised, it will disintegrate within 24 hours. The corpus luteum will carry on producing progesterone for a couple of days, but it then disintegrates. The drop in progesterone causes the lining of the womb to begin to break up, and it is shed as the period begins and we are back to day one of the cycle again.

When am I most likely to conceive?

We tend to have it in our heads that we are most likely to get pregnant around day 14 of our cycle, but in fact, that's not particularly useful unless you have a regular 28-day cycle. Ovulation occurs roughly 14 days before your period arrives, no matter how long your cycle is, and it is the first half of the cycle, when the egg is growing and maturing, that causes most of the variation in menstrual-cycle length. This means that if your cycle is 35 days long, you will ovulate somewhere around day 21, whereas a woman with a 25-day cycle will ovulate around day 11. It may sound confusing, but you just work two weeks back from your period to work out when you have ovulated. If you have a regular cycle, you can use this to tell when you are likely to be ovulating in future months.

It is obviously far more difficult to pinpoint ovulation if your periods are not always regular. In general, if you are having sex every two or three days, you are likely to be hitting your most fertile time, and this will maximise your chances of conception.

Fertility specialists estimate that women are usually fertile for between six and eight days of their cycle, up to and including the day of ovulation. You are most likely to get pregnant if you have intercourse a couple of days before you ovulate, as this will give sperm time to be ready and waiting in the fallopian tubes for an egg.

Ovulation prediction kits

Kits for predicting ovulation have become very popular with women trying to conceive, as they seem to offer some certainty and reassurance that ovulation has occurred. They work by measuring the surge of hormones that triggers ovulation using a simple urine test. In theory, this allows you to time your most fertile moment, just before ovulation, and make sure you always have intercourse when you are at the peak of your fertility.

However, there are a number of problems with this. The surge in hormones is what sets ovulation off, and it is quite possible to have a surge without actually releasing an egg, so the kits can give a false sense of security. We have seen that there is a fairly short window of opportunity for an egg to be fertilised once you have ovulated, which means you will be most likely to conceive if you have intercourse a couple of days before ovulation, and before a test would show positive.

The other problem is that ovulation prediction kits are most commonly used by women who don't have regular cycles and who want to find out when they are ovulating. The tests usually contain enough test sticks for five days, which may not be sufficient for women who have irregular periods. You may end up needing a number of kits to get it right, and this can become an expensive business. So, the kits are least likely to be a real help to the women most likely to use them.

Temperature charts

Compiling temperature charts used to be one of the main ways to check whether a woman was ovulating, as it was discovered that progesterone, which is produced during the second half of the cycle, causes your body temperature to rise. For many years, keeping a temperature chart was suggested to any woman trying unsuccessfully to have a child. The idea is that you take your temperature as soon as you wake up every morning, and plot it out on a chart. The chart should show a rise at ovulation, when progesterone makes your temperature increase, and it should then remain slightly higher for the rest of the cycle until your period starts, when it will drop. You can buy special extra-sensitive thermometers and ovulation charts to help you monitor this, but there are many other reasons for your temperature to fluctuate, and current medical opinion does not recommend keeping temperature charts, as it is no longer believed they can predict ovulation reliably.

Cervical mucus

It is probably not something you are used to discussing, but your cervical mucus can be a useful indicator of when you are at your most fertile. This method of checking ovulation is sometimes called the Billings method, named after John and Evelyn Billings, the two doctors who developed it.

If you stop to think about it, you will probably be aware that sometimes you have a fairly thick, white cervical mucus, whereas at other times it is watery and transparent. This is due to changing hormone levels in your body. If you watch out for changes, you should find that there are a few days in the middle of your cycle when the mucus looks almost like egg white and there is much more of it. This is sperm-friendly fertile mucus. It allows the sperm to swim freely, and indicates that you are about to ovulate. Immediately after ovulation the mucus becomes thick and dry again, acting as a barrier.

Some women find it relatively easy to judge their most fertile time by a quick mucus check, indeed they may be aware of it anyway, but not everyone feels comfortable with this. Apparently, the best way to test it is by inserting a finger into your vagina and circling it about to collect some mucus to inspect, but the faint-hearted may prefer to use a piece of loo paper to wipe the entrance to the vagina and then examine that. If you're really interested, you can start a fertility chart and plot your mucus changes. For the technically minded, there is even computer software that allows you to tap in your daily temperature, cycle length and mucus condition to work out a detailed cycle analysis.

You can also feel your cervix itself, assuming you know exactly where to feel. It is at the top of your vagina, and should feel firm, low and closed for most of the month. At ovulation, it should feel open, raised and soft. You may need a bit of practice with this one, though.

The right time

Of course, it is vital that you're having intercourse around the time of ovulation, but if you have a rough idea of when that might be, and make sure you have sex every two or three days around that time, you are going to be hitting your most fertile period. Some couples get very concerned about timing intercourse, but all the evidence suggests that this can just make you stressed and have a negative effect on your sex life. In general, more sex means you are more likely to get pregnant, and making sure you are getting enough around the time you think you are most fertile is better than trying to pinpoint specific days.

Preventing pregnancy

Women spend most of their fertile lives trying not to get pregnant, and primitive methods of contraception have been around for thousands of years. Women have inserted pastes, fruit acids or other dubious mixtures into the vagina, and used lemons or sponges as vaginal barriers. Some of these methods may have worked to a degree, but there were still many unwanted pregnancies. By the eighteenth century there were male condoms made of animal intestines, and Victorian women used an early form of rubber diaphragm, but it is only relatively recently that women have had easy access to reliable methods of contraception.

We tend to think that as soon as we have unprotected intercourse we will get pregnant, but our choice of contraceptive can have an effect on our future fertility. It may take a while for a normal menstrual cycle, and normal fertility, to be restored after using some methods of contraception.

Barrier methods are one of the simplest forms of contraception, which work by stopping sperm getting into the womb to meet an egg. Barrier methods include male and female condoms, which have the added advantage of helping to protect against sexually transmitted diseases, and the cap or diaphragm, which fits over the neck of the womb and stops sperm getting past. It is possible to get pregnant the moment you stop using barrier methods of contraception as they have no effect on your future fertility.

Spermicides are put in the vagina before intercourse and can kill sperm. They may help protect against some sexually transmitted diseases as they can also kill bacteria and viruses, but the downside of this is that they can cause irritations and allergic reactions. Spermicides are not very reliable when they are used as the sole method of contraception, but it is possible to get pregnant as soon as you stop using them.

Combination oral contraceptive pills contain synthetic oestrogen and progesterone. They work by stopping ovulation, thickening the cervical mucus to prevent sperm penetrating it and by thinning the lining of the womb to stop a fertilised egg implanting. There are no long-term links with infertility after taking the combined oral contraceptive pill, but it can take two or three months for the menstrual cycle to return to normal. Some women do experience longer-term difficulties conceiving after taking the pill, but these are usually related to underlying medical problems or age, rather than the pill itself.

The contraceptive patch works the same way as the combination pill, but instead of swallowing the hormones in a pill, you stick them to your body in a sort of square plaster. Hormones are then slowly released through the skin. It can take a few months for your periods to return to normal when patches have been used.

The progesterone-only pill is also commonly known as the mini-pill. It contains synthetic hormones similar to progesterone, and works by thickening the cervical mucus and thinning the lining of the womb. Some progesterone-only pills stop ovulation in some women too. One common side effect of the progesterone-only pill is irregular or unpredictable bleeding. There is also an increased risk of ovarian cysts, and if you do get pregnant while on this pill there is a small risk of having an ectopic pregnancy, which can cause fertility problems in the future. It may take a few months for your cycle to get back to normal when you stop taking the pill, but generally women on the progesterone-only pill return to normal fertility fairly quickly and longer-term problems are usually to do with underlying medical problems or age.

The contraceptive injection is an injectable synthetic progesterone, which lasts for up to three months. Some women do suffer a loss in bone density with this method of contraception, leading to concerns about osteoporosis, and it can cause weight gain and irregular bleeding. After the last injection, it may take six months for the drug to leave the body entirely and for the menstrual cycle to return to normal. For some women, it can take more than a year for their fertility to be restored after using the contraceptive injection, but the length of time it takes to conceive afterwards does not seem to be related to the length of use.

The contraceptive implant is a small flexible rod, thinner than a matchstick, which is inserted under the skin in your upper arm. It releases a synthetic progesterone and is effective for up to three years. It can cause weight gain, and irregular or heavy periods, but once the implant has been removed your normal cycle should return quickly.

The intrauterine device (IUD) is a T-shaped plastic device that is fitted inside the womb. It contains copper, which immobilises sperm, and the IUD also makes it harder for eggs to meet sperm or for fertilised eggs to implant. Once the IUD is removed, your normal fertility usually returns immediately, but IUDs are associated with an increased risk of infection, which can cause infertility, and on very rare occasions they can damage the womb itself. Although the IUD is a highly effective contraceptive, it cannot prevent an egg implanting in the fallopian tubes, and so for the tiny percentage of women who do get pregnant while using one there is an increased risk of ectopic pregnancy, which can in turn lead to tubal damage and infertility.

The intrauterine system (IUS) is another T-shaped device that has to be fitted inside the womb, but it works differently from an IUD and is sometimes referred to as a hormonal IUD. The IUS releases synthetic progesterone, which thins the lining of the womb, thickens the cervical mucus and can sometimes prevent ovulation too. The synthetic hormone in the IUS can lead to a delay in re-establishing a regular menstrual cycle but normal fertility should return fairly quickly.

The morning-after pill is an emergency contraceptive that should be taken within 72 hours of unprotected intercourse, although it is most effective within the first 24 hours. It is similar to normal combined or progesterone-only pills, but has higher doses of synthetic hormones, and it works by stopping or delaying ovulation or implantation. It can disrupt your next period, but doesn't have any other effect on your future fertility.

Sterilisation should only be contemplated if you are absolutely certain you will never want it reversed. It involves cutting the fallopian tubes and tying them up or sealing them, or blocking them by clipping them with rings or clips. Reversing sterilisation is a difficult and expensive process, which is not always successful. It usually entails chopping out the section of tube that has been damaged, and joining the ends back together. If the ends of the tubes have been tied or sealed, it can be even harder to reverse the operation. Anyone who gets pregnant after they have had a sterilisation reversal has a higher chance of an ectopic pregnancy.

For women who have a partner who has had a **vasectomy**, which involves cutting the tubes that carry sperm from the testes into the penis, the prospects are not much better. Vasectomy reversals don't always work and this is a delicate surgical procedure with huge variations in success rates. In general, no more than half of vasectomy reversals are successful, but this seems to depend on how long it is since the original vasectomy was carried out. If it is less than three years, there is a higher chance of success. In some cases, there are sperm in the semen after a vasectomy reversal but the sperm motility is poor, and they are not capable of getting a woman pregnant.

Natural family planning means you avoid having intercourse on your most fertile days, and you can buy natural family-planning kits if you want to use this method. They may monitor saliva, use urine tests or computerised thermometers, combining your body temperature, which rises when you ovulate, with other information about the length of your cycle. When you are trying *not* to get pregnant, the advice is that there are about ten days of the month on which you should avoid having intercourse. This errs on the side of caution as women who are trying to get pregnant are usually told there are eight days at the most on which they can conceive.

You can, of course, save money and do your natural family planning by charting your own cycles, but it usually takes a few months to recognise all the signs your body gives out when you ovulate, and it is only really easy to do this if you have pretty regular cycles. The advantage of using natural family planning if you're going to want to get pregnant later is that you will already have worked out precisely when you are at your most fertile during each cycle. It could be said that this is one form of contraception that may have a positive effect on your chances of getting pregnant in the future. The disadvantages of this method are that it involves diligence and commitment, and can be unreliable.

Chapter two

Finding the Right Time

For some women, finding the right time to have a baby is about finding the right circumstances. You may have reached an age where you feel you can't leave it any longer, you may have found the partner you plan to be with for the rest of your life, you may have got to a point in your career where you've achieved what you wanted or you may just feel financially secure and settled.

For others, trying to find the right mindset is more of a barrier to having children than the circumstances. Making a conscious decision to start a family can seem a monumental step, particularly as we feel we have more choice in the matter than previous generations, and are aware of the lifestyle changes it will involve.

Feelings about motherhood

Our ideas about how we see our lives progressing, and whether being a mother is important to us, are often shaped at an early age. Women may have very strong and certain feelings about this, or may be unsure where and how motherhood will fit into the lives they want to lead.

Knowing what you want

Motherhood is an essential part of how some women see their future, and it may be something you have always known you want in your life. You may not be wondering whether you are going to have children, but simply when you are going to get around to it. Women who feel this way may still want to wait for the right circumstances, but having a family is not something they are prepared to compromise on, and they will put themselves through whatever it takes in order to try to achieve this goal.

Motherhood doesn't hold the same attractions for everyone, and there are many women who are equally adamant that they don't ever want to have children. They may be put off by the responsibilities of having a family, and prefer instead to keep their careers, lifestyles and finances intact, or they may relish the freedom of being child-free. Making the decision not to have children is not always easy in a society that can seem to revere the family. Women who choose to be child-free may find that people assume they must be career-orientated hard-nosed types who don't have time for children in their lives, and they may feel pressured by others who cannot understand their decision.

'I think there's a lot of peer pressure. There's this expectation that it is just something that happens when you've been with someone for a long time and it is an established

relationship. I never ask people why they do have children, but they always feel they have to ask me why I don't.'
Sara, 44

The traditional pattern

Not all women have such definite views one way or the other when it comes to procreation, and the decision to have a child does not always involve any particularly deep thinking or longing. For our grandmothers, and indeed many of our mothers, having a baby was not something to be pondered and discussed. Starting a family was just what was expected once you were married.

Today, many couples dispense with marriage, but settling down with the right partner is usually followed at some point by discussions at least about starting a family. With so many more choices, having babies is no longer an inevitability, but the majority of couples may still expect it to happen sooner or later once they are in a stable relationship.

'I didn't even think about children until I got married, and then I assumed that at some point we would want a family. I never thought about how much I wanted it. I just assumed it was a natural progression and that I ought to want it.'
Julie, 40

Leaving it to chance

Although most of us have had the need for effective contraceptive use drummed into us from our teenage years, research suggests that as many as one in three pregnancies are unplanned. Although some of these pregnancies may be the result of contraceptive failure, far more are due to risk-taking. Women who had been feeling slightly ambivalent about motherhood may discover that getting pregnant unintentionally takes the element of choice away. Although some may opt to terminate the pregnancy, many decide that they want to keep the baby, particularly if they had been hoping to have children in the not too distant future.

It can be hard to make the decision to start a family, and you may never feel that the time is absolutely right. Couples who are dithering about making the commitment sometimes leave it to chance by being less careful about contraception. Although they may not be actively trying to have a baby, they may not be trying particularly hard not to have one either.

Making a commitment

Women's lives today are not always child-friendly. Our jobs often involve working long hours or lots of travel. Enjoying a social life, going out with different partners, seeing the world and having some life experiences can all feel more immediately important than starting a family. We may want to achieve some of our other goals in life before we are ready to think about having babies, and this means that more and more of us are well into our thirties before we seriously consider motherhood.

For young professional couples who may have spent many years enjoying their freedom and their lifestyles, starting a family can appear to be a huge life-changing step. Once you start analysing the pros and cons, you may never feel you are at precisely the right point in your life.

Financial security is very important to some couples, who need to feel that they are settled and have enough money before making a commitment. Others may want to wait until they have a home with enough space for a child, or until they've got that promotion or pay rise they've been anticipating. The reality is that we could always be more financially secure and settled, have a larger home or have got one step further in our careers, and there is always an excuse when we are not entirely sure. For a generation accustomed to having so much choice, it is not an easy decision.

'I think it's quite a scary thing to do. In a way, you never feel ready, and we both had periods of thinking we'll make the decision and start trying, and then complete panic that we had made that decision. I think it is hard, particularly for our generation, because we are used to being quite selfish really and we do see it as giving up stuff. I think for our parents it was just more automatic.' *Rachel, 31*

What influences the decision?

For each individual, there may be a number of different factors that finally convince us we are ready for children. They may come from within and be related to our particular circumstances, or there may be external influences which lead us to the conclusion that the time is right to start trying for a baby.

Catalysts

Sometimes it is an outside event that alters your perspective, and can suddenly make you think that you are ready to make the decision to have children. It can be a relatively obvious matter of a friend or relative getting pregnant or having a baby that makes the idea more appealing, but the catalyst can come from anywhere and can be set off by any event that makes you take stock of your life and think seriously about your future.

'I'd never wanted children. It just wasn't important. I was very much into my career, getting on in life. I had other things to do. Then my granddad died, and I started wondering whether it was something to think about.' *Corinne, 36*

Your age

Age is often the key factor in making the decision to start trying to have a family. We know that we get less fertile as we get older and that we risk not being able to have children if we leave it too long, but at the same time most of us want to have enjoyed some child-free time before we submerge ourselves in the responsibilities of family life.

If you know you want children, and particularly if you feel you'd like more than one, your age is not something you can choose to ignore. Although many women do get pregnant in their late thirties and early forties, by this age we are well past our peak fertility. It would be wonderful if there were no time restraints on female fertility and if concerns about being able to cope with small children were the only potential worry of starting a family in our forties. If you know you want a child eventually, your awareness of the ticking of your biological clock may be more important than anything else in pushing you towards motherhood. Many women do find that at a certain point they suddenly feel ready to have children, but this may happen to one woman in her twenties, and another in her late thirties and is likely to be affected by your circumstances.

'I started to think about my biological clock when I was 29. I'd been with my partner then for nearly nine years and I was very aware that I was getting near to 30, and that while my husband-to-be could take all the time in the world to make his choices, I couldn't.' *Siobhan, 41*

Your job

Fitting a family around your career can be difficult. We no longer believe that we need to choose between a career and a family, but we may have concerns about being side-lined at work, or having to reduce our options once we have children. Finding the right time to have a baby often involves some kind of compromise on the work front. Women who get pregnant in their early twenties may build successful careers once their children start school, whereas those who wait until they are heading towards the top of their career paths may find it easier to take a break as they are already well established. Most women think about starting families somewhere in between these two points, and it is not always the easiest time from a work perspective.

Some jobs, and some employers, are far more family-friendly than others and offer good maternity benefits, plenty of time off and even the opportunity of returning to work part-time or working flexibly. The downside of arrangements like these is that they may involve stepping sideways, or even backwards, on the career ladder, but that can seem a price worth paying if you are trying to juggle work and childcare. Some women manage to fit children around their careers very successfully, and having a family may be just one of many priorities, but, for others, becoming a mother is always going to be the most important role.

Your relationship

The decision to start trying to have a baby can be particularly difficult if your partner is less keen to make a commitment. Men are largely free from time constraints on their fertility, and although research suggests that there may be some age-related decline in male fertility, they are unlikely to feel the same pressure to have a child sooner rather than later. A woman in her late thirties will be aware that she is cutting it fine if she wants a family, particularly if she intends to have more than one child, whereas her male counterpart may feel safe in the knowledge that waiting another five years is unlikely to make a great deal of difference to his chances of becoming a father.

It can be tough if you feel ready, or if you are worried that time is running out, and your partner wants to wait. Women in this situation often feel they are being forced to make a choice between having a child and staying with their partner. This dilemma does put an end to some otherwise happy relationships, or alternatively can leave women resenting the fact that they feel they are wasting their remaining fertile years waiting for a partner who isn't ready to commit.

It is not always the female partner who is rooting to start a family. Women have to carry babies, give birth and breastfeed, and sometimes it is the woman who is reluctant to try to get pregnant, as she may be keenly aware that the advent of children means her life will change far more than her partner's. Women still bear the brunt of childcare responsibilities in most relationships, and may be worried about the sacrifices they know they will have to make.

Most couples do eventually come to some kind of agreement when one of them is keener to start a family than the other, but it is important to make sure that you are both happy with your decision, as having children, or choosing not to have them, will affect the rest of your lives.

'I never wanted kids from a young age. I didn't have that maternal instinct. My husband is more traditional. I would have left it later if he hadn't wanted kids, but I'm glad he pushed me into it when we got married. I could potentially have resented losing my freedom if I'd had kids earlier, but now I am ready.' *Mikaela, 32*

Waiting for the right partner

Perhaps the most important factor of all in finding the right time to have a child is finding the right person to build a family with. In our twenties, our priorities may be more focused on our careers and social lives than on finding the right partner to settle down with, but as we get older, and more aware of our biological clock, the pressure to meet the right person can become intense. Most of us have grown up with the expectation that we will meet someone first and then start a family, and for women in their thirties who feel ready to have a child, the lack of a suitable partner can be the major stumbling block.

In the past, women in this position might have felt their only option was to settle down with the first vaguely acceptable man who came along, but we may be less prepared to make that kind of compromise today. Women are used to being financially and emotionally independent and to taking responsibility for their own lives, and may not be willing to accept the idea of a less than ideal relationship just because it will give them the opportunity to have a child. Using donor sperm, it is possible for a woman to have a child without having a man, and this is a way ahead that more women are actively considering.

'I had the option to go out and find myself a bloke but that's easier said than done, and also very wrong to get into a relationship because you want children and then split up a few years later, or get drunk and have a one-night stand. I didn't want my six-year old to say, "Who is my daddy?" and to shrug my shoulders and say, "I don't know – some bloke …" The option of being childless is very sad, and I live in an age where I have the choice and the technology to prevent that.' *Mary, 41*

Lesbian couples and motherhood

Whereas once their sexuality might have stood in the way of motherhood, it no longer poses the same kind of problem for lesbian couples, who can use donated sperm to start a family. The lifestyle factors involved in finding the right time to have children, feeling settled in a relationship, being financially secure and the restraints of the biological clock are exactly the same, but a lesbian couple must also make a decision as to which of them will carry the baby. This may be based on age and work circumstances, as well as considering which of them is most keen to experience pregnancy and birth.

'I always assumed that I would have children. I came out as a lesbian when I was 18 or 19. That was just about the time when there was a lot of publicity about lesbian mothers. I never thought there would be a contradiction between the two things.' *Naomi, 39*

Finding what's right for you

For all women, single or with a partner, gay or straight, finding the right time to have a child involves taking into account a whole series of considerations based around our situation, circumstance and expectations. Having children is no longer an automatic step, and although having more choices may have made our lives richer, it has also made the decision-making process more complicated.

The time may never feel absolutely ideal, but an awareness of our biological clock can help crystallise our thoughts. Despite all the advances in reproductive technology, we have to accept that we may not be able to leave it as late as we would like, and our age may be the crucial decision-making factor for many of us. Finding the right relationship is often key too, although it is no longer unusual for women to sidestep this, particularly if they feel time is running out. Feeling secure and settled, being at the right point in your career, having the right home or the right salary may all influence your decision, but we have to remember that each of us will have her own interpretation of her circumstances, and must make her own decision about when the time is right.

Chapter three

How Late Can I Leave it?

It's an unfortunate fact that the female reproductive system has been rather left behind by the changes in women's lives during the last century. We expect to be able to finish our education, establish our careers, settle down with the right partner and have some degree of financial security before we think about having babies. We want to wait until we feel we are ready to start a family, but this may mean our bodies are past their fertile best.

Although there have been recorded cases of women conceiving naturally in their early fifties, and of far older women getting pregnant after fertility treatment with donated eggs, these are rare exceptions. More usually, women will find that their fertility is in decline by the time they reach their forties. It is true that many older women get pregnant naturally and without any difficulty, but for others putting it off until their forties, or even their late thirties, may turn out to be a gamble they have lost.

We are so accustomed to being in control of our fertility that it's easy to forget that this is a relatively new-found freedom. It wasn't until the introduction of the oral contraceptive pill in the 1960s that women gained real control over their reproductive systems. Society had changed, women had attained a greater degree of equality in education, the workforce and the home, but our fertility has remained one area in which we are far from equal. We are born with our lifetime's supply of eggs, whereas men can continue producing sperm throughout their lives, and although they experience some age-related decline in their fertility, it is far from absolute. Men may still be fathering children when they are drawing their pensions, but most women run out of viable eggs during their forties.

We are sometimes lulled into a false sense of security about our fertility, and having spent many years preventing pregnancy when we don't want it, we assume we will be able to exercise a similar level of control when we do want to get pregnant. For some women, this may turn out to be the case, but others will find conceiving a child much more difficult.

'Education should actually inform women that they shouldn't leave it too late. In schools it's all about safe sex and contraception and you mustn't have a baby. Maybe we should be a bit pro-baby as well, preface the safe sex with, "Don't forget, if you want to have a baby, you should do it at a sensible age."' *Susan, 34*

The biological clock

The female biological clock begins ticking when we are born. We lose eggs from our ovaries throughout our child-hood, and by the time we reach puberty and are able to conceive, our egg store has already been depleted. Our fertility declines throughout our adult lives, but every woman's biological clock runs at a different rate. One woman may get pregnant naturally in her early forties, while another may run out of eggs in her twenties, experiencing a premature menopause.

> 'People don't understand that your biological age can be very different to your reproductive age. At 29, my reproductive age was 42 and that's a big problem. People say they're going to delay it because they aren't ready and they think if they leave it until they are 38 or 39 that will be their reproductive age, but it's not necessarily the case.'
> *Rachel, 35*

As recently as the 1970s the average age for having a first child was 25, but now most women have reached their late twenties by the time they give birth for the first time and many more delay motherhood until they reach their thirties. By this age, most of us are approaching the end of our optimum fertility, and there is a growing awareness that delaying motherhood may lead to fertility problems, as the biological clock starts to speed up as we get older.

The endless discussion in the media about the way female fertility declines with age could lead some women to seek medical solutions too quickly for what may be little more than a natural age-related delay in conception. However, there is also an assumption that assisted conception offers women a safety net when nature lets us down. In fact, fertility treatment is much less successful as you get older, and it cannot turn back the biological clock.

'When we got married there wasn't as much in the media about fertility as there is now. I wish that what's in the media now about the fact that you're much more fertile when you're younger and that having a baby isn't something that happens automatically had been higher profile then. I would have come off the pill on the wedding night.'
Lana, 37

Assessing your own fertility

So, is it possible to tell whether you're one of those women who will be able to get pregnant easily if you put it off until you are older, or whether you really ought to start trying as soon as you can if you want to have children eventually? Unfortunately, it is impossible to give any kind of definitive answer, but there are some indicators that may help you assess whether you are more at risk of having problems.

Fertility indicators
Are your periods regular?
Women who have regular periods are more likely to be ovulating, and less likely to be entering the perimeno-

pause (the term given to the years which lead up to the menopause itself). If your periods are irregular or absent, this can suggest problems with your hormones, and may also be a symptom of polycystic ovary syndrome: a condition that can prevent normal ovulation. Very heavy bleeding is sometimes a symptom of fibroids, benign tumours that grow around the womb and which can affect your fertility.

The length of cycle is also relevant. Anything between 25 and 35 days is generally considered normal, and if you have a regular cycle of this kind of length you are more likely to be ovulating.

Have you had a sexually transmitted disease?

Women who've had chlamydia and gonorrhoea are at greater risk of having fertility problems, as is anyone who has had pelvic inflammatory disease, which is not always sexually transmitted. Many women with these infections experience no symptoms at all, and yet if they are left untreated they can lead to scarring in the ovaries or fallopian tubes, tubal blockages or ectopic pregnancy. Those most at risk of sexually transmitted disease are younger, sexually active women who have had multiple partners and who don't always use condoms.

Have you had surgery in your pelvic area?

If you have had surgery to remove an appendix or ovarian cyst, or any other kind of surgery on your womb, ovaries or fallopian tubes you may be more at risk of infertility, as this can leave scarring that may block the fallopian tubes.

Are you very overweight or underweight?

Being naturally slim or on the rounded side is not going to stop you getting pregnant, but weight problems can have serious consequences for your fertility. Women who are underweight often stop ovulating, and those who have a history of eating disorders will often find that their periods are affected. Equally, very overweight women may have ovulation problems, which make them less likely to conceive.

Doctors use the Body Mass Index, or BMI, to calculate whether people fall outside the healthy weight ranges for their height. If you want to work yours out, you divide your weight in kilograms by your height in metres squared (that's your height in metres multiplied by itself). If your maths isn't up to it, you can find lots of easy calculators on the Internet to work it out for you, where you just type in your weight and height. The general rule is that a BMI of over 30 or under 20 could affect your chances of conceiving.

BMI is a rather blunt instrument and doesn't take account of an individual's frame or muscle, which weighs more than fat. It is possible for a super-fit athlete to fall into the overweight bands by being extremely muscular, but this isn't an excuse that will apply to most of us. Generally a very high or low BMI does suggest we should look at our diet and levels of exercise.

Do you have endometriosis?

Endometriosis occurs when tissue similar to the spongy womb lining is found elsewhere in the body, usually in the pelvic area around the ovaries and fallopian tubes. The most common symptoms are pelvic pain and irregular or heavy periods, although some women are unaware that they have the condition. Many women with endometriosis get pregnant without any problems at all, but it is estimated that between 30 and 40 per cent of sufferers have difficulty conceiving.

Do you smoke, take recreational drugs or drink too much alcohol?

These can all have adverse effects on your fertility, and make you more likely to miscarry or to have problems with the pregnancy when you conceive. If you are a smoker, try to give up, and if your partner smokes, get him to stop too. Smoking, and even passive smoking, has been clearly linked with reduced fertility. Heavy alcohol consumption, binge drinking and recreational drugs can all have an impact on your fertility too.

Do you lead a healthy lifestyle?

Eating healthily and taking regular exercise will help keep your body in good physical condition, which will maximise your chances of conceiving. You don't have to sign yourself up for a punishing fitness regime to reap the benefits of exercise, particularly if you tend to be a bit of a couch potato. All you need is regular gentle exercise to increase your physical strength and stamina, and it can also improve your general well-being. Trying to ensure you have a healthy diet is often difficult when you lead a busy life, but if you can manage to eat healthily you are more likely to be getting the essential nutrients, vitamins and minerals that help your reproductive system to work properly.

How old was your mother at her menopause?

If you know that your mother had a very early or late menopause this may have a bearing on your own fertility. It is believed that there is often a genetic link when it comes to the biological clock, and that your own menopause may be early or late depending on your mother's experience.

Home testing

You can now buy tests, from a pharmacy or online, that aim to help you assess your own fertility. They check your hormone levels to try to give you an idea of the quality and quantity of eggs remaining in your ovaries, known as the ovarian reserve. Some use a simple urine test that can be done in the privacy of your own home, and give an instant result. Others involve a blood test that has to be sent away to a laboratory for analysis.

The tests work by measuring your levels of FSH (follicle-stimulating hormone), which is an indicator of the ovarian reserve. When the ovaries are full of good-quality eggs, your body doesn't have to work particularly hard to ripen and release them, but as the eggs get older and their numbers decline, the body has to produce higher levels of FSH to help them on their way. Some tests also measure inhibin B and anti-Mullerian hormone, (AMH) as low levels of these hormones may suggest a poor ovarian reserve.

Although these hormone levels can give some indication of ovarian reserve, they often fluctuate from cycle to cycle. One test alone may not give a particularly accurate picture of what is happening in your ovaries, and for this reason some of these products include two tests so that you can check your initial findings. The tests can be expensive, and if you are really worried that you may be approaching the menopause, you may be better off going to see your doctor and having tests done professionally.

It is also important to remember that a test result indicating a good ovarian reserve doesn't give you the green light to assume that you will get pregnant if you wait another two, or three, or five years before you try to have a baby. Although they may be useful at alerting you to a problem with your eggs, the tests can't assess other aspects of your fertility. It is quite possible to have a good outcome and yet to find that there may be other factors that could make it difficult for you to get pregnant naturally.

Fertility by decades

The way women think and feel about their fertility is often dependent on their age, and the experience of getting pregnant is coloured by the stage in life at which we experience it. In our teens we tend to have a carefree attitude towards our fertility, and pregnancies at this age are often unplanned and unprepared for, whereas by the time we reach our early forties, a pregnancy may have taken some time to achieve and can seem more precious, but it may be overshadowed by concerns about possible risks and problems. Just as a woman's fertility changes with age, so does her experience of pregnancy and motherhood.

Getting pregnant in your teens

Teenage pregnancy is often seen as an indicator of government failure to provide adequate education and accessible contraception to young people. Although we are all aware that getting pregnant when we are older carries medical risks, we may be less aware that there are medical risks for teenagers who get pregnant too. Teenage mothers are more likely to develop anaemia and high blood pressure, to go into labour prematurely and to have a low-birth-weight baby with a greater risk of health problems.

Teenage mothers may face other social difficulties that can cause problems, along with the fact that they may not access regular antenatal care early in their pregnancies. There are also the obvious hardships of attempting to finish an education, establish a career and become financially secure while caring for a young baby.

'I was 17 when I got pregnant. We wanted it to happen but we hadn't thought it through properly. We were both really happy, but after a few weeks we were thinking, oh my God, what have we done? I've always wanted to be a mum, and I don't regret it now. By the time my son is 18, I am going to be 36, so I'll still have most of my life ahead of me.'
Fran, 20

'I was just 18 when I found out I was pregnant. It was a big shock. I went to my GP to talk about having an abortion, but that's as far as it went. Changing my mind was the best thing I ever did. It was hard; there's that whole stereotype about young mums scrounging on benefits and stuff, and we were determined not to be like that. I started my nursing training when my son was two, and we've bought our own house.' *Emma, 27*

Getting pregnant in your twenties

Biologically, this is the ideal time to have a child. Women in their twenties are twice as likely to conceive as women in their late thirties. Your body is young, you probably have a good egg supply, you are more likely to get pregnant quickly and less likely to miscarry or have pregnancy-related problems.

However, in just about every other way, this may seem far from the best time to have a child. We still feel young in our twenties, we want to enjoy life, to travel and have fun, and we don't want to be tied down with responsibilities. We may be in full-time education and want to find a job we enjoy, to establish a career, sort out our finances and make a home for ourselves before thinking about having babies. Perhaps more vitally, many women in their twenties have yet to find a partner they feel they would like to settle down and have a child with. So when our bodies are at their reproductive peak, many of us are far from ready to make the most of this.

'I was 26 when I got pregnant. I think I'd always imagined I'd have children one day, but it certainly wasn't planned. I did miss out on some things. I don't think I have the financial stability that I would have liked ideally, and I do think perhaps I could have lived my life more fully.' *Louise, 30*

Getting pregnant in your thirties

Many women today are finally ready to have a child in their

thirties. This is often an age at which women feel settled and start to think of motherhood after working hard to establish a career and waiting to meet the right partner. Our thirties are also the most crucial period of change in our fertility. At the start of the decade most women are still very fertile with a good chance of conceiving, but by the time you reach the age of 35 you are only half as fertile as you were at 25. As you approach 40 your fertility declines sharply, and while some women conceive perfectly easily at 38 or 39, others will have problems.

Although you need to be aware of the age-related changes in your fertility, it is also important to remember that many women today have their first child in their thirties without any difficulty, and there are some advantages to being a 30-something mother once you have got pregnant. You are likely to have a healthier lifestyle than your younger counterparts, to eat more healthily and nutritiously and to take more exercise. All of these will benefit your baby as you go through pregnancy. You are also likely to be more tolerant of the changes pregnancy and motherhood will bring to your life, and to be a more confident parent.

'By the time you get to your thirties, you know who you are and feel a bit settled. When you've met the right person, then go for your family. Rear your children between 30- and 40-something, and then you can claim some life back again.'
Siobhan, 41

'I'm trying to accept that I'm older and I'm doing everything I can to try to offset my age. It depresses me to even use

the word, but you are in a race. Every month when you get your period, the finishing line gets further and further away.'
Lana, 37

Getting pregnant in your forties

By the time you reach 40, your fertility is in sharp decline. On average, a naturally fertile woman who doesn't use contraception will have her last child at around this age. At 40, most women are still having regular periods, but once you reach 45, the menstrual cycle will usually start to become irregular. The menopause may not follow for another six or seven years, but your fertility is compromised for some time before this.

The risk of miscarriage also increases in older woman. It is thought that up to half of pregnancies in women over 40 may miscarry, but this often happens early and goes unnoticed. There is also a higher risk of problems for the baby, and women in their forties have a greater chance of having a child with Down's syndrome or chromosomal abnormalities.

During your forties the number of follicles in your ovaries is declining rapidly and you not only have fewer eggs but their quality is also affected. It is thought that the ageing hypothalamus in the brain may play a role here too, as the female reproductive system is very finely tuned, and even a small irregularity can send it out of synch. Although your womb is also getting older, this seems to be less of a problem where maintaining a pregnancy is concerned, as women in their forties who use eggs donated from a younger woman are often successful.

Being pregnant can be more difficult for older women. Mothers in their forties are more at risk of high blood pressure and pre-eclampsia, and may find pregnancy exhausting. However, babies born to mothers in their forties have some advantages as their parents are likely to be more confident and may have waited a long time for a baby, who will be much loved.

'I've only just turned 40, and the build-up was dreadful. Forty and no children ... I go to the park and I see all these girls that are my age or younger with all their kids packing up a picnic, and I want to be a part of that. I want that in my life.' *Andrea, 40*

'I was 41 when I had my daughter. On balance, it's different, but it wasn't any harder for me being a mother in my forties. Being older, you do have less energy, but I think you make up for it in other ways. You've got more patience and you're more accepting.' *Tanya, 44*

The menopause

The menopause marks the end of a woman's reproductive period of life. It normally occurs between the ages of 45 and 54, and on average a woman will be about 51 when she goes through the menopause.

The menopause begins with a phase known as the perimenopause. During this time the number of follicles left in the ovaries decreases, and the body produces less oestrogen and progesterone. The follicles no longer respond so well to the hormones FSH and LH (luteinising hormone) sent from the pituitary so the body starts to make more of these. This is why FSH levels are sometimes used to check the ovarian reserve and assess how close a woman is to the menopause.

As the FSH and then LH levels slowly rise and the body produces less oestrogen and progesterone, women may start to be aware of menopausal symptoms. These usually begin several years before the menopause itself, and include irregular periods, hot flushes, night sweats, sleep problems, dry skin, hair loss, headaches, mood changes and decreased sexual desire. About 70 per cent of women experience some kind of symptoms, whereas other fortunate types manage to get through the whole thing with no symptoms at all.

Eventually the ovaries give up trying to release mature eggs and the woman's periods stop completely. A woman reaches the menopause when a year has passed since her last period. Once this has happened, there is no longer any chance of pregnancy using her own eggs.

Premature menopause

Some women go through the menopause many years, even decades, before they would expect to, and this brings their fertility to an early end. It is known as premature menopause, or premature ovarian failure, and it can happen when women are still in their teens or twenties. The causes of premature ovarian failure are often unclear, but there are hereditary links, and if it happened to your mother, it is more likely to happen to you.

Women are often unaware of what is happening unless they are trying to have a child, as experiencing menopausal symptoms at an early age may be totally unexpected. Sometimes it is only during fertility investigations that the problem is discovered.

'When I asked my mum what age she'd gone through the menopause and she said she had completely finished by the age of 41 as three generations of my family had, alarm bells went off. I went to the doctor and they said it was very likely that I would have a hereditary premature menopause as well.' *Susan, 34*

Pregnancy after the menopause

The cases of women giving birth in their late fifties and sixties that hit the headlines always involve the use of another woman's eggs. Egg donation was first developed in the 1980s as a way of treating women who had problems producing their own eggs, and it is not only used for those with premature ovarian failure or poor egg quality, but also for women who have a history of genetic disease, who have had to have their ovaries removed for medical reasons, who have not responded to previous fertility treatment, or who are just older.

It seems that although the biological clock stops us producing viable eggs as we get older, it doesn't affect our wombs in the same way. So women who have already been through the menopause and stopped producing their own eggs can successfully give birth if they use eggs from a younger donor. In theory, this means that women who are happy to use donated eggs can wait as long as they like to have a baby. In practice, most clinics set age limits for egg donation and will not treat women who are past their late forties or early fifties. There are few doctors in the world who are willing to offer headline-making treatment to women in their sixties.

Egg freezing – an insurance policy?

'I looked at freezing eggs, but it just wasn't an option because of the money it would cost. I was told that the success rates were low, but if you're in the position that I was in and it is your last option, then you just accept that it is a last resort. You think, I'll give it a shot – but basically I couldn't afford it.' *Susan, 34*

Frozen eggs have been touted in the media as the solution to all women's age-related fertility problems. It has been suggested that any woman who knows that having children is really important to her should consider freezing some of her eggs while she is young to allow her to delay motherhood until she is ready.

It sounds fantastic. You freeze a batch of eggs in your twenties when they are still young and fresh, you build your career, buy your home, meet the right man and maybe wait to have your babies until your forties. The problem is that egg freezing is still a new science. Until very recently most eggs didn't survive the freezing and thawing process, as they are much more fragile than embryos. New techniques are being developed, and some clinics are reporting much better outcomes with frozen eggs, and are also freezing ovarian tissue as an alternative. However, egg and ovarian-tissue freezing are expensive procedures, involve invasive medical techniques and are not particularly likely to succeed. They may offer hope to women who know their fertility is likely to be compromised by cancer treatment, or who are expecting to go through a hereditary premature menopause, but they can't be used as a guarantee of a child in the future.

Chapter four

Boosting Your Fertility Naturally

Whether you have decided you're ready to get pregnant and want to improve your chances of conceiving, or whether you're more interested in preserving your reproductive system for as long as you possibly can, there are some things you can do that may help. Although we may not be able to halt the pace of our biological clock, which was set at birth, we certainly can make sure our lifestyle choices aren't speeding it up.

Where your choices matter

We may be able to influence our fertility by making some quite simple changes to our lives. How much attention we pay to our health, what we eat and drink, and what we do at work and in our spare time can all make a difference.

Smoking

If you are a smoker, giving up is one of the most important things you can do to help increase your chances of getting pregnant and improve your fertility. Women who smoke often take longer to conceive, and smoking can affect your ovarian reserve, reducing egg quality and quantity. Women smokers are twice as likely to have fertility problems as non-smokers. On average, women who smoke reach the menopause two years earlier than non-smokers, and they are more likely to have an early menopause. One study has suggested smoking can shorten a woman's reproductive life by ten years. What's more, it's not just your own smoking that can affect your fertility – if your partner smokes, that can cause problems too. Women who live with a smoker have been shown to take longer to get pregnant.

The dangers of smoking once you get pregnant are very clear-cut. Women who smoke expose their babies to tar, nicotine and carbon monoxide. Smoking reduces the amount of oxygen and the level of nutrients that reach the baby, and pregnant women who smoke increase their risk of having a miscarriage. Their babies are more likely to be underweight, premature or to die in infancy. There is a link between smoking and breathing problems in young babies, and with cot death.

Many women who smoke intend to give up once they get pregnant, and it makes sense to cut out cigarettes as soon as you start thinking seriously about trying to have a baby. The good news is that if you do stop smoking, after just a year of abstinence your chances of conceiving are thought to be as good as those of women who have never smoked.

Drinking

Moderation here, as in all things, is the key. You should certainly be drinking less than the recommended upper limit of 14 units a week for women, and it is often advised that women who are trying to conceive should give up alcohol altogether. This may be a good idea, but for some women it is not an entirely realistic proposition, particularly if it ends up taking some years to get pregnant. Most of us enjoy an occasional social drink with friends or a glass of wine with a meal, and if you can restrict yourself to this, it is not likely to damage your fertility. Research suggests that women who drink more than five units of alcohol a week take longer to get pregnant, and the general advice if you're trying to conceive is to limit yourself to one or two units once or twice a week.

It is clear that excess and binge drinking have a negative effect on female fertility, and can lead to irregular periods or anovulatory menstruation (which means you still have periods but you are not actually ovulating). It is not just the alcohol itself that causes problems, but also the impact it has on your overall health. Women who drink too much often don't sleep or eat properly, and it can affect your sex life. If your partner is drinking more than three units a day, this can reduce his sperm quality too.

When you're trying to work out whether you may be drinking too much, you should be clear exactly what constitutes a unit of alcohol. Generally a unit is one level of spirits, a half-pint of beer or a glass of wine. However, many bars and restaurants now serve wine in large glasses, and these usually contain at least two units.

Alcohol can also increase the risk of miscarriage once

you get pregnant, and one of the biggest dangers to the baby if the mother drinks during pregnancy is foetal alcohol syndrome, which can cause mental handicap

Caffeine

It has been claimed that just one cup of coffee a day can reduce your fertility by half, but the evidence is not consistent when it comes to the link between caffeine consumption and infertility. Consuming very large quantities of caffeine is not a good idea anyway, and the crucial level seems to be around 300mg a day, which means your caffeine intake could possibly cause problems if you drink more than three or four cups of coffee, six cups of tea or eight cans of cola in a day. One study found that women who drink more than five cups of coffee a day were at greater risk of miscarriage. Despite the conflicting evidence, it makes sense not to drink too many caffeinated drinks if you are trying to lead a healthy lifestyle.

Recreational drugs

You wouldn't if you were pregnant, so don't if you're trying. Recreational drugs may be a part of many women's social lives nowadays, but they can reduce your fertility and increase your chances of miscarriage. Marijuana, often seen as the acceptable face of recreational drugs, can be particularly damaging to both male and female fertility.

It is worth noting here that if your male partner uses anabolic steroids, he may be seriously impairing his chances of having a child. Anabolic steroids can have some pretty horrid effects on the male reproductive organs, causing testicles to shrink and sperm production to be reduced or to come to a complete halt. Although these effects can usually be reversed once the drugs are stopped, this is not always the case if high doses of anabolic steroids have been taken for some time.

Prescription drugs

You should check whether any prescription or over-the-counter drugs that you use on a regular basis might have an effect on your fertility. Some non-steroidal anti-inflammatory drugs, such as Ibuprofen, can affect ovulation. Thyroid replacement hormones, antidepressants, tranquilisers and asthma medication have all been linked to fertility problems. For men, some antibiotics, antihistamines, antimalarial drugs, blood-pressure treatments and arthritis drugs may cause problems. If you, or your partner, are taking any medication on a regular basis, it is worth checking that it isn't going to affect your chances of getting pregnant.

Weight

Women's weight and eating habits are often tied up with our emotions and how we feel about ourselves. Although we are constantly warned about the growing obesity problem in developed countries, we also see girls becoming concerned about being 'too fat' and dieting at alarmingly young ages. Female fertility is affected by extremes of weight, but there is a wide scale in the middle where both slim and curvy women fall within perfectly healthy weight ranges.

Although stick-thin models may rule the pages of

fashion magazines, being really skinny is not going to help you get pregnant, and the chances are that many of these women we often think of as 'ideal' are not fertile. When a woman has too little body fat, it causes her periods to stop, and you can't get pregnant if you aren't ovulating. It will also be much harder to conceive if your body is deprived of vital minerals, vitamins and nutrients.

Women who have eating disorders may not always realise that they are putting their fertility at risk. It is common for women with anorexia to stop ovulating, and bulimic women often develop polycystic ovary syndrome, which affects their fertility.

At the other end of the scale, obesity also has an impact on ovulation. Fat cells produce oestrogen, and excess weight can lead to raised oestrogen levels, which may prevent ovulation by suppressing the pituitary gland and the release of FSH. Women who are overweight are also more likely to have polycystic ovary syndrome. If your partner is very overweight, this could reduce his fertility by affecting his sperm quality.

Weight may affect the outcome of fertility treatment, and there is a lot of debate as to whether women who are very overweight should be offered treatment. It is claimed that assisted conception is less likely to work for obese women, as they do not respond so well to the drugs, and they are also more likely to have problems in pregnancy.

Losing weight is often enough to reverse the fertility problems associated with obesity. However, when women are unhappy because they can't conceive, they may resort to comfort eating, and this can turn into a vicious circle.

'I'm an emotional overeater, so having so much pressure put on to lose weight because of this was really impossible. I found it incredibly difficult because the more upset I was, the more I wanted to eat. In the last few months, because we're going for IVF and I know we're spending all this money, I've found the strength and got my weight down to what it is meant to be.' *Lisa, 32*

'I was very overweight. I wasn't particularly unhealthy, but I desperately wanted to lose weight. I'd tried every diet under the sun, I'd tried exercise, I'd tried eating healthily, I'd tried absolutely everything. I started a diet where you have nutritional food packs instead of food. It is a very drastic diet, but you do it under the supervision of your doctor. I had six stone to lose, and in three months I had lost two stone.' *Clare, 34*

Exercise

Apparently most of us don't get enough exercise. It helps maintain our bodies in good working order, as well as increasing fitness and strength. It has just as important a role in keeping us emotionally balanced, reducing stress and making us feel relaxed. It is often beneficial for those who suffer from depression, anxiety or insomnia. There are long-term health benefits too, as it can help prevent high blood pressure and heart problems.

It is hard to find the time to exercise when we're leading busy lives, and sometimes there simply isn't space to fit in a visit to the gym or the swimming pool, but if you don't take any exercise you'll end up feeling tired and sluggish, and your body will not be in peak form for conception.

Don't launch into some manic exercise regime if you usually spend your spare time in front of the television. Try to find a form of exercise that you can fit into your day, start gently and do something you actually enjoy. That way you're far more likely to stick at it.

As always, you can have too much of a good thing, and women who do huge amounts of exercise can have problems with ovulation. We are talking about extremely vigorous exercise here, and it isn't an excuse to avoid a brisk walk around the park, as this problem mainly affects female athletes who are in regular training.

Diet

Eating properly means your body gets the fuel it needs to function at its best. We're all pretty well versed in the rules of healthy eating now – a balanced diet with lots of fruit and vegetables, making sure you have sufficient protein, carbohydrate and unsaturated fat (that's the sort you get in olive oil, seeds and fish rather than in meat and dairy products). We are familiar with the fact that we should try to eat fresh produce wherever possible, avoiding too much fast food and processed stuff, and that we should eat oily fish and drink lots of water.

When you're busy, perhaps working late or away from home a lot, it can be hard to find time to cook, or even to make sure you're eating something vaguely nutritious. Office canteens tend not to offer much in the way of fresh fish, brown rice and organic vegetables, and sometimes when you are really pressed, it can be hard to find time for lunch at all. It is simply not possible for many of us to eat the perfect diet every day, but you can make a difference if you try to be more aware of what you consume, and to choose the healthiest options you can.

The food many of us eat is also full of additives, and you may want to try to cut down the amount of processed convenience foods you consume and consider using organic produce. If you're not sure about something, read the label. Sometimes surprisingly few of the ingredients listed on ready-meals are actually recognisable as food.

'We didn't drastically change anything to do with our diet because we've always eaten quite healthily anyway. I bought everything organic, and I drink more water than I used to, but I didn't start buying anything else other than that. You hear of all these weird and wonderful things, but you have to be careful because you are vulnerable.' *Sandra, 41*

With diet, as with everything, a balance is essential. You will come across lots of advice about food and fertility, which may involve cutting out all kinds of things entirely, from dairy produce and red meat to sugar and wheat, but for most of us this would not be a particularly enjoyable experience. What's more important, we probably wouldn't stick with it for very long. It is far better to make less dramatic changes to your diet that you know you will be able to live with.

'Nutritionists say to cut out all dairy and all wheat and all this … You might try it once, but to be honest I think the most important thing is to remain sane, and try and stay calm about it. I found stopping all your pleasures in life at a time when you are quite stressed actually has a detrimental effect. I was stuffing down chocolate bars, and drinking a few glasses of red wine, and really enjoying it.' *Helena, 34*

Vitamin supplements

In recent years, there has been a surge of interest in natural solutions to fertility problems, and holistic fertility clinics have been springing up all over the place. Understandably, they have proved popular with couples trying to conceive who are keen to do everything they can to improve their chances of having a baby. Many of these clinics recommend supplements to help with vitamin and mineral deficiencies, which it is believed may be at the root of some male and female fertility problems. Zinc, selenium, vitamins E and C are often recommended, but you do need to be careful if you are taking lots of different vitamin supplements, as the cumulative effects of taking large doses of individual vitamins are unclear.

'They gave us a ton of vitamins and minerals – huge amounts of them. When I did my second IVF, the doctor asked me what medication I was on, and I said I was taking tons of vitamin C. He said it was far too much and I shouldn't be doing that. So after that I thought I wouldn't do that again, I'd focus on trying to drink less and be fitter instead.' *Debbie, 44*

If you are worried that you may be lacking in some essentials, it is perhaps better to take a daily multivitamin. One study showed that women going through IVF and taking a daily multivitamin had considerably better outcomes than those who didn't take the multivitamin. In an ideal world, we would be getting all the nutrients and vitamins we need from our diet, but in reality this isn't always the case and taking a daily multi-vitamin is certainly not going to do any harm.

The one individual supplement you should make sure you take if you are trying to get pregnant is folic acid, as it helps prevent neural-tube defects in babies developing in the womb. Some multivitamins designed for women who are pregnant or who are planning to conceive contain additional folic acid. Once you are pregnant, you should not take any other supplements unless you've checked with your midwife or doctor.

Your lifestyle

Many of us lead hectic lives that leave little time for relaxation. We may dash to work in the rush hour, spend long, often stressful, hours at the office, drink coffee to keep ourselves going, then too much alcohol after work, arrive home too late to cook supper and find it difficult to sleep. Inevitably our bodies suffer when we don't take care of them, and it is important to try to maintain some kind of balance in your life.

There are conflicting opinions as to whether stress may play a role in causing infertility, but it is clear that when women go through stressful times their menstrual cycle is often affected. Sometimes there is an increase in the level of prolactin a woman's body produces when she faces a crisis, and it can stop ovulation altogether.

When you are trying to get pregnant without success, this causes a great deal of stress itself. Telling women who are trying to conceive that they should stop being so stressed about it is not particularly helpful, as much of their stress may be caused by their condition.

'There was a year when I was just totally stressed out about not being able to have children. I knew I needed to relax, and I had been relaxed when we first started trying, but then the pressure starts. From starting out feeling fairly chilled about the whole thing, two years had gone by before we started to panic. Then there was a year where it was all I thought about.' *Isla, 35*

The longer a woman tries unsuccessfully to get pregnant, the more worried and stressed she becomes. People will tell you to relax, go on holiday, forget about it. Everyone seems to know one of those couples who had a baby as soon as they decided to adopt or to give up on fertility treatment. The reality is that it doesn't work for most of us. Even so, it is worth trying to find some time for yourself in your life. Exercise is an excellent way of reducing stress, as is yoga or massage, aromatherapy or meditation. Even just walking instead of taking the car or bus can make all the difference to how you feel.

Your job

We may suspect that long hours in a stressful job have an effect on our fertility, and if you're trying to get pregnant unsuccessfully, you may start wondering whether your job could be partly to blame. The idea that women make a choice between a career and a family is often still thrown at anyone who has a successful career and is trying unsuccessfully to conceive.

Women can find it difficult to cope with their jobs when they start going through fertility tests and treatment, but how any individual deals with this depends on the level of support and flexibility they are offered. A sympathetic employer can make all the difference. Some women find it helps to reduce their working hours when they are having fertility treatment, but for many others this is simply not a realistic proposition.

'I was very lucky. The company I work for was absolutely brilliant. My boss and colleagues were incredibly supportive. I changed my hours, and everybody arranged their meetings around my schedule. In my department at work, myself and another woman had done IVF and two of the guys were going through it as well. It was amazing. Just by being open and honest about it, we managed to find ourselves a fantastic support network.' *Nic, 33*

It is perhaps after repeatedly unsuccessful attempts at treatment that work can become really tough. If you're going through lots of treatment cycles fairly close together, you may need more time off work than is sustainable, and some women do stop altogether for a while, whereas others find work provides a useful distraction from their fertility problems.

Environmental hazards

Every day we are exposed to chemicals and toxins, but there is little clear evidence as to how they may affect our reproductive systems. Part of the problem is that there are just so many potentially damaging substances in everyday products like household cleaners and pesticides, solvent-based paints, additives and preservatives. Although individual chemicals or toxins may have been tested and declared safe, we don't know the cumulative effects of being exposed to so many all at once. It is clearly impossible in the twenty-first century to lead a life free from pollutants and chemicals, but you can try to limit your exposure by cutting back on your use of these products in your home.

There may be more specific hazards in the workplace. We know that exposure to radiation and pesticides can have a harmful effect on the human reproductive system, and there are suggestions that other substances could inhibit fertility, although there is not always clear scientific evidence. Agricultural workers may be exposed to pesticides, and wood workers, smelters, anaesthetists, nurses, pharmacists and dental assistants may all come into contact with chemicals that may affect their fertility. Lead, mercury, nitrous oxide and formaldehyde have been linked with reduced fertility, and if you are exposed to any of these on a daily basis, or have concerns that other chemicals you use at work may be affecting your fertility, you should talk to your doctor.

Chapter five

I'm Not Pregnant Yet

You've decided to try to have a baby. You've thought about it, you've had the discussions and now you're ready. You've thrown away the contraceptives, and you've started trying. At first, it's great ... you're full of optimism and ready to go, you're thinking of names and planning how you'll decorate the baby's room. When your period arrives the first month, you're not too bothered. After all, you knew it might not happen right away. Then another month passes, and another, and period after period after period, and you find yourself starting to worry ...

How long should it take?

When you've spent most of your adult life trying not to get pregnant, it is only natural to assume you'll conceive as soon as you allow it to happen. Most of our sex education centres on the idea that unprotected intercourse will lead to unwanted pregnancies, and it never occurs to most of us that we might find that we can't get pregnant when we want to.

In fact, less than a third of couples conceive straight-away, and it is perfectly usual for it to take a few months. Around 75 per cent of women will conceive in the first six months of trying for a baby, rising to about 85 per cent after a year. These are the average figures for all ages, and on the whole women who are older are more likely to take longer to conceive. For those between the ages of 35 and 39, there's just a 60 per cent chance of getting pregnant after a year of trying. Although this does clearly illustrate that women become less fertile as they get older, it doesn't mean that all women over 35 will necessarily have problems. The majority of women of this age who want a baby will still get pregnant without any medical help. In general, the longer you have been trying to conceive without success, the less likely it is to happen, and couples who have been trying for a baby for more than three years have around a 3 per cent chance of conceiving during each cycle at the most.

'We grow up being told that if we miss one contraceptive pill, that's enough to get pregnant if you have unprotected sex. We believe that we've created a situation of choice, where we can choose what we want to happen to our bodies and when we want it to happen, and, of course, nature plays tricks on us.' *Siobhan, 41*

When should I seek help?

Making the decision to get medical help is not always easy. Some women prefer to leave it to nature for as long as they possibly can before they get embroiled in the whole business of tests and medical interventions. Others start worrying that something may be wrong fairly quickly, and want to rule out any potential problems after just a few months.

Age Your individual circumstances will determine how soon you should think about seeing a doctor, and once again, your age is probably the most crucial factor. If you're in your twenties, you may want to leave it 18 months before you approach your doctor, but women who are over 30 are usually advised to seek help after a year. If you are over 35, it makes sense to start investigations even sooner, after about six months, as if you do find you have problems and end up needing treatment, it is less likely to work once you reach your late thirties or early forties.

Medical history Your medical history is also important here. If you've had an ectopic pregnancy in the past, if you know you have fibroids or have had any previous gynaecological problems, you should see your doctor sooner rather than later. Women who have had tubal or pelvic surgery, pelvic inflammatory disease or any sexually transmitted infection should also consider seeking help more quickly.

Menstrual cycle Your menstrual cycle is relevant, as an unusual cycle can indicate problems with ovulation. If you don't have periods, if your cycle is less than 25 days or longer than 35 days, or if it is very irregular, this can suggest that you may not be ovulating normally and you should talk to your doctor.

Male conditions There are some male conditions that may also make it advisable to see a doctor earlier. If your partner has had mumps, this can affect the testicles and cause problems with sperm production, and if he had to have an operation as a child to help his testicles drop, this may also be relevant. Men who have had a sexually transmitted infection in the past may be at risk, and should consider ruling out any sperm problems earlier on.

Health Your general health can make a difference to how quickly you get pregnant. If you are very overweight or underweight, if you smoke, take drugs or drink a lot, you may be making it more difficult for yourself. Of course, many women do all these things and manage to conceive perfectly easily, but if you are starting to worry about not getting pregnant, you may want to make some lifestyle changes before you start testing your fertility.

Frequency of sex It may sound very obvious, but you're not going to find it easy to get pregnant if you aren't having enough sex. A woman's most fertile time is generally thought to be about two days before she ovulates, but it is usually possible to conceive during the six days leading up to ovulation. Once an egg has been released, there is a relatively short period of time in which it can be fertilised, so you are most likely to get pregnant if there are sperm ready and waiting. If you are having sexual intercourse three times a week, you are unlikely to be missing this window of opportunity.

Seeing a doctor for the first time

It is perfectly normal to feel awkward about approaching your doctor to discuss the fact that you aren't finding it easy to get pregnant. Sometimes admitting this to your doctor entails a shift in attitude from feeling vaguely concerned that things aren't happening to accepting that there may be something wrong. Many couples feel apprehensive about this, and it may help to know that problems getting pregnant are the most common reason apart from pregnancy itself for women between the ages of 20 and 45 visiting their doctor.

Most doctors are sympathetic to fertility problems, but some couples do feel that they don't get the attention they need and deserve. If you have been trying to conceive for some time and are starting to get upset about the fact that you're not getting pregnant, this is a problem that deserves to be taken seriously. If your doctor tells you to go away and keep trying when you've already spent more than the recommended amount of time doing just that, you may want to consider seeing someone else.

'After about a year when nothing had happened I started to think that it wasn't right. We started off by going to the doctor but he wasn't very good. He didn't take us seriously and he said to just give it time. It all seemed very slow at first. They say you're just being impatient and that things will happen when they happen, which is fine if it does, but sometimes there's a problem and it needs sorting.' *Ann, 44*

It makes sense to take your partner with you for the first visit to the doctor, as any potential fertility problem could lie with either of you. Many women end up going alone to their first appointment, partly because they may be worried more quickly than their partners, and aware of the time limits on their fertility.

'My husband thought I was worrying too much that I wasn't getting pregnant. He kept saying it would happen eventually. In the end I went to the doctor about something else, and mentioned I was worried because we'd been trying for a baby for months and nothing had happened. The doctor said he might as well do some tests right away. I think my husband was surprised when I came home with a sperm sample pot for him after going to the doctors about painful periods.' *Carol, 45*

At the initial visit, the doctor may look back over your medical history and carry out basic physical examinations and blood or sperm tests to make sure there is no obvious problem. Sometimes they may prefer to refer you on to a specialist right away.

Fertility clinics

Your doctor can either refer you to your local hospital for tests, or to a specialist fertility clinic. Although a local hospital may be more convenient, and have a shorter waiting time to see a gynaecologist, it is usually worth going straight to a fertility specialist. They will deal with you and your partner as a couple, and will be able to carry out more thorough tests and offer a wider range of treatments. Sometimes your doctor will suggest which clinic you should go to, or will make the referral without any consultation, but if it is left up to you to choose a clinic, this can be a difficult decision to make.

'You put so much trust in the medical profession, but when it comes to fertility it's not that I don't trust people, but it is a business and it's a bit different to going in and having an operation on your appendix. It's a big money-making industry, and you have to go into it with your eyes open. It's very hard to do that when you are emotionally fraught, but I say to people, do your research.' *Rachel, 35*

Not all fertility clinics offer every type of treatment, some see many hundreds of patients every year and employ dozens of doctors, whereas others are much smaller; some may specialise in particular areas of infertility and there can be huge variations in success rates. So how do you decide where to go? If you have a choice, it is worth doing some research, and there are some key factors that may influence your decision.

Location

The location of the clinic is probably the most important thing to consider. There is little point in discovering what appears to be a perfect clinic if it is based at the other end of the country. It may be that there is only one clinic situated anywhere near your home, which leaves you with little choice. In other areas, there may be an abundance of fertility clinics and making a decision can be difficult.

You need to remember that you could end up having to make fairly regular visits to the clinic if you have treatment, and a journey that seems fine for an occasional appointment can rapidly become unmanageable when you are having to make frequent trips to and fro. Sometimes it is possible to have certain tests or treatments carried out at a local hospital under the auspices of a specialist clinic further away, but not all centres offer this kind of facility.

'We ended up going to a clinic which is a 150-mile round trip. If I had my choice again, I'd have chosen something closer to home. I wasn't sure what was involved, and hadn't realised I'd be there every second day for scans. Whenever I had to go for a scan, I had to get the day off work.'
Elissa, 32

Location is obviously important, but you should also feel confident that a local clinic can offer what you need. If you go to your local treatment centre purely because it is convenient and don't consider any other factors, you may end up questioning your choice when you are further down the line.

Treatment

The treatment a clinic can offer is equally important. Not all clinics offer every type of fertility treatment. Some specialise, or may have a reputation for being particularly good at treating certain problems. You should check what a clinic offers, and how many patients they treat. You may find that some clinics have restrictions and set an age limit for treatment, or may not treat those who have specific complications. Make sure you are aware if this is going to be the case.

'Sometimes it is a bit of luck to find the right person because there is no list of who is the best specialist for each individual thing. At the end of the day, it's like any problem. Even if you've got a plumbing problem or whatever, it is getting the right person to do the job. You can get a lot of cowboys who will try, but you need to get the right person who will give you the right information and be honest with you.' *Ann, 44*

Success rates

Success rates may be the clearest indication you have of how well a clinic does at any particular treatment. These are published regularly and make it easy to compare how well a clinic is doing, but they should be taken with a degree of caution.

As the success rates usually involve the number of live births after particular types of treatment, they are inevitably rather out of date by the time they are collated, and the rates can vary hugely from one year to the next. Success rates are also very dependent on the patients who are being treated. If a clinic is seeing a lot of patients with complex medical conditions, a large percentage of older women, or those from lower socio-economic groups who have poorer general health, this will be reflected in the success rates. You should try, as far as you can, to find out what chances of success the clinic would have for a woman of your age with similar fertility problems.

'I did quite a lot of research into the clinics and I think that was the best thing I did. I didn't know how much they varied at the beginning. I've seen so many of our friends who've gone though IVF at really useless places. It's a combination of finding a fit for you, getting the best you can. No one is really there to help you. You have to help yourself.' *Helena, 34*

Cost

The cost of both tests and treatment can vary widely. If you are going to be paying for your care, make sure you have a breakdown of exactly what each type of treatment or test will cost. Sometimes there are hidden extras, and patients can find they end up paying far more than they expected when they get their bill. You should check exactly what is and isn't included in any figures you are given.

Clinic staff

The clinic staff can make a huge difference. You may want to know whether it will be possible to see the same person every time you go to the clinic or whether you will end up seeing whoever happens to be on duty. Some patients like to know whether there is a choice of male or female doctors.

'There was no continuity of care. It was a different person every time I had a consultation, every time I had a scan. Every time you walked in you didn't know who you were going to see. You never felt you were able to say to them, "Since we last spoke I've been doing this or this," because you'd never seen them before. It was very frustrating.' *Nicol, 33*

Recommendation

Personal recommendation is always helpful if someone you know can recommend a clinic, but remember their circumstances may be different from yours. Just because someone else has been successful at a particular clinic, it doesn't necessarily follow that you will too.

Waiting lists

You may want to check whether there is a long waiting list for an initial appointment and for any treatment you may need. Some clinics see patients as soon as they are referred, but others may take a while to see you, and may have long waiting lists for treatment.

'We feel we have been failed in our area. The waiting list for treatment is currently three years at our local clinic. They don't carry out lots of basic tests, they put everyone on clomifene and send you away for six months, and then they put you back on this long waiting list. It's not something you want to hang about with, so that seemed really pointless.' *Debbie, 29*

Atmosphere

It may sound a ridiculous thing to worry about, but the atmosphere in one clinic may just feel right to you, whereas another doesn't. This is very much a personal thing. Large clinics often have the highest success rates, but some patients complain that they are daunting and impersonal. At a smaller clinic, people know who you are and you can get to know them. This can be more relaxed and relaxing, which is an important factor for some women. Sometimes when you are having treatment, it is the little things that can really make a difference to how you feel.

'We went to see one clinic, and as soon as we walked in I had a gut instinct that it was the right place to be. They just put me at ease. It was a very small unit, and it didn't feel like a factory. They were interested in my welfare and in our situation. They listened to you as an individual.' *Lulu, 39*

One common complaint patients have about fertility clinics in larger hospitals is that they are often situated in the women's health departments and may be right next door to the maternity unit. This can be distressing, and it is something you may want to consider.

'The clinical care was very good, but the environment was not good. The waiting room was connected to the maternity unit, so my husband and I would be sitting there surrounded by pictures of babies and notices about breast-feeding. It was just so insensitive.' *Jane, 45*

Counselling and support

Counselling should be offered at any clinic that carries out fertility treatment. You may feel you don't need counselling, but it can really help with the emotional trauma of not being able to have a child, and is often beneficial if you end up having fertility treatment. It is worth checking whether counselling is included in the cost of any treatment. You may also want to know whether there is a counsellor on site, or whether you would be expected to see someone elsewhere.

Some women feel uneasy about seeing a counsellor, as if it is an admission that you are not coping, but counselling can make all the difference to how you feel about your situation, particularly if you find someone you like and trust.

'We had no support from family, and friends were limited, so we had to revert to the counselling that the hospital provides, and it was wonderful. It really was an outlet for us. We went very regularly, every four weeks, for a long time. It was just nice to be able to talk about our problems.' *Emma, 38*

Lesbian couples and single women

Single women and lesbian couples may find that not all clinics will treat them, although the situation has changed considerably in the last few years and there is much less prejudice about this. Attitudes do vary from clinic to clinic, and if you have a choice it may be worth gauging the reception you will get before coming to a decision.

'I did phone around clinics and some were quite blatant, and actually quite rude, just saying they didn't deal with lesbians. At some points I did feel like the door was being slammed in our face, but we did find clinics that would deal with us.' *Sarah, 28*

Reputation

The vast majority of fertility consultants and clinics are highly reputable and their services are closely monitored to ensure they maintain good standards, but some patients do feel unhappy with their treatment. There should be a proper complaints procedure in place at every clinic if you are concerned about something, and if you have any doubts about the treatment you are being offered, you should make sure they are answered before you agree to go ahead. Really thorough research is undoubtedly helpful if you have a choice of clinics.

'I looked up IVF clinics, went to visit all the different doctors and as soon as I came out of the consultation I wrote a list of the pros and cons of each doctor. I put down everything from the smallest detail, things like how I felt when I walked into the clinic and whether I liked the receptionist, all the prices and that kind of thing, everything I could possibly drag out of my head. I just weighed them all up.' *Debbie, 44*

Telling other people

Some couples tell their friends and family as soon as they make the decision to start trying to have a baby, which means they will realise fairly soon that things aren't going according to plan. If you haven't told anyone you're trying, you may start feeling pressured by people asking you when you're going to get round to it, and sometimes it is easier just to be honest and say it is taking longer than you hoped, which will usually put an end to the conversation. It is common not to want to tell people you've been trying unsuccessfully, as this may feel like admitting something is wrong when you haven't really come to terms with that fact yourself.

How you feel about telling people depends a lot on your relationships with individuals, whether they are members of your family or friends. Some people don't understand and don't know how to deal with it, whereas others are very sympathetic. It can be helpful to have a friend to confide in if you are feeling upset, but people don't always react in the way that you would hope, and one of the most common complaints is that other people just can't seem to say the right thing. You are probably quite sensitive, and although your friends and family may be trying to be helpful, it won't always feel that way.

'You can't talk to anybody about it because they just don't understand. Unless you've been through it you haven't got a clue. It can be difficult but you just put up with it and put on a brave face.' *Nikki, 35*

Support groups

Some fertility clinics have their own support groups, or you may find a local group that is part of a bigger network. There are a number of support organisations dealing with specific fertility problems and some of these have local groups that may hold occasional meetings. Support groups sometimes meet at local hospitals, at members' houses, or just get together at a local bar. Groups do vary considerably. Some of the well-established support groups are very organised and lend books and videos, arrange social events or visiting speakers and may even produce their own newsletters.

It can seem daunting to turn up at a meeting with a roomful of strangers when the only thing you have in common is the difficulty you are having getting pregnant, and support groups may not be suitable for everyone, but many people do find them really helpful.

'I think a support group is a wonderful thing. I did have people I could talk to, but you reach a point where you think you are going to bore everybody, and you don't want to keep moaning all the time. In a support group, people understand and they don't judge you.' *Gillian, 30*

For some women, the thought of joining a support group can be one step too far, as it can seem as if you are accepting your infertility, which you hope will be short-lived, as a real long-term problem.

'I looked on the Internet for local groups and I couldn't decide whether I wanted to meet people in the same situation or whether I really didn't at all. I had second thoughts about doing anything like that because it made it more real. I almost didn't want to be part of a group who were infertile women because I didn't want to accept I was one of them.' *Rachel, 31*

Support groups used to be the only way of getting in touch with others with the same problem, but now many people prefer not to have to go out and face what they fear could be an awkward meeting with a group of strangers. The popularity of traditional support groups has declined in recent years as the Internet has taken over as a way of getting in touch, and some support groups find they are more successful when they arrange casual meetings in bars or cafés, rather than the more formal hospital setting.

Internet support

Fertility support on the Internet has become hugely popular, and there are any number of online support networks that will help you to find other people who have the same fertility problem, who are going through the same tests and treatment, and who may even be at the same clinic. There is always someone to talk to, help is there whenever you need it, and you don't need to leave your home to access it. Many women find themselves online friends, or 'cycle buddies', who are going through treatment at the same time, and find it really useful to be able to discuss their experiences as they happen.

'There were six or seven of us who were starting a cycle at the same time and we went through the whole month on a forum talking it through. It was incredibly helpful. It was small things like the first time you have to inject yourself. It was really useful to go on and read somebody else saying it wasn't as bad as they thought. It made it much less scary.' *Nicol, 33*

When you first start using the fertility websites, it can be hard to work out what on earth people are talking about. If someone tells you they and their dh have been ttc for four years, have just been through their 2ww after IVF and had a BFN, you may be completely confused. This means they and their partner (dh – dear husband) have been trying to conceive (ttc) for four years, have just been through the two weeks of waiting to find out whether they are pregnant (2ww) after having IVF and have been unsuccessful (BFN – big fat negative). Fortunately, most sites have a page translating all the abbreviations and you may find yourself whizzing back to them a lot at first.

Although many women find Internet support absolutely invaluable, you should bear in mind the fact that postings on message boards are from other patients, and some of the advice and information they give may not be medically accurate. At the same time, for a patient's-eye view of treatment, they are incredibly useful.

For some women, even Internet support feels too intrusive, whereas others don't like the idea of talking intimately to people they don't know. In those circumstances, the information produced by national support networks and books about infertility can prove a godsend.

The main benefit of any kind of support wherever you prefer to find it is the realisation that you are not the only woman living with this, that there are many others out there who are going through exactly the same thing and experiencing the same emotions.

Chapter six

What Can Go Wrong?

The female reproductive system is incredibly complex, and one in six women find they have some difficulty getting pregnant when they want to. It isn't always easy to pin down where things are going wrong because subtle imbalances in our bodies can interrupt the finely balanced chain of events that sends mature eggs down the fallopian tubes to the womb. It is sometimes only once we find we have problems getting pregnant that we start to appreciate what an amazing process it is.

There is still much that we don't understand about female fertility and why some embryos implant successfully and others don't. Many women never discover why they can't conceive, as there are parts of the process doctors can't check and monitor. However, there are some common problems that may stop you getting pregnant.

Hormonal problems

Around 20 per cent of fertility problems are caused by

ovulation disorders. Women may not be releasing eggs at all, or may not be ovulating regularly. Sometimes, the ovaries don't produce mature follicles and the eggs can't develop properly. Ovulation can be disrupted at any point along the route that passes messages from the brain to the ovaries, and any kind of irregularity may stop eggs being released normally.

Polycystic ovary syndrome

Polycystic ovary syndrome, also known as PCOS, is a very common cause of female fertility problems. More than 20 per cent of women have polycystic ovaries, where small cysts are found just below the surface of the ovaries. These cysts are actually follicles that haven't developed properly. For most women, the cysts are not accompanied by any other symptoms and they still ovulate regularly, but some women also have other symptoms of PCOS.

If you have PCOS you will usually have irregular, infrequent or absent periods. This means you are not ovulating regularly, and your body may not be releasing mature eggs at all. The syndrome is often associated with weight problems, and about a third of women with PCOS are overweight. Women with PCOS are often told to try to get their weight down as this can improve their fertility, but unfortunately it can be harder to lose weight if you have PCOS.

Not everyone who has PCOS is overweight, and it is quite possible to have the syndrome and be very thin. PCOS often affects women who have eating disorders, and if you have bulimia you have a high risk of developing PCOS, even if your weight is normal.

There are some other signs that can accompany PCOS. You may have unwanted facial or body hair, and skin problems such as oily skin or acne. Some women also experience hair loss, or thinning hair. Women who have PCOS usually have imbalances in their hormones, and may produce higher than normal levels of testosterone. They may also have high levels of insulin, the hormone that regulates blood-sugar levels.

'I think I have had PCOS all my adult life. When I was 16, I came out in the worst acne of my life. I had very heavy periods, was very hairy, had dandruff … all the PCOS signs. I had blood tests and a vaginal scan, and they confirmed it was PCOS.' *Sarah, 34*

Raised prolactin levels

Ovulation can also be disrupted by raised prolactin levels. Prolactin is a hormone that helps prepare women's breasts for milk-production after childbirth, but high levels in women who are not pregnant can affect the normal hormonal balance. The symptoms of raised prolactin levels are irregular or absent periods, and you may also have a milky discharge from your breasts. Stress can cause prolactin levels to rise slightly, as can some types of medication.

Premature menopause

Also known as premature ovarian failure, premature menopause is usually defined as the onset of the menopause before the age of 40. It is thought that around 2 per cent of women have a premature menopause.

It is often not clear what makes the ovaries stop functioning normally at what ought to be the most fertile period of a woman's life, but it sometimes has genetic or chromosomal causes. A premature menopause may be the result of cancer treatment or autoimmune disorders.

If your mother had an early menopause, you are more at risk of this yourself, and if this is the case and you've already been trying to get pregnant unsuccessfully, you should seek medical advice sooner rather than later. Women who know they may be predisposed to a hereditary early menopause will usually be referred for treatment quickly if they are trying unsuccessfully to conceive, but doctors may be less willing to address the concerns of single women in this position who are worried about their future fertility. Once a woman has reached the menopause, the process is irreversible however early it may happen, and the only way to get pregnant is by using another woman's donated eggs.

'They did all the blood tests and they showed that my hormone levels were at the level of a 42-year-old. At the time I was 29. They said I wasn't going into the menopause right there and then, but the likelihood was that I would go into an early menopause and not have any eggs, or the eggs might be bad quality.' *Rachel, 35*

Endometriosis

A common condition, endometriosis is named after the endometrium, the spongy womb lining that develops every month. Endometriosis occurs when tissue similar to the endometrium starts growing outside the womb. It is most commonly found around the ovaries, womb, bowels or bladder. It is thought that 15 per cent of women may suffer from endometriosis, and many of them conceive naturally without any problems, but in some cases it can affect fertility.

The most common symptom of endometriosis is pain, either in the abdomen, the lower back or the pelvis. Some women find they have painful, heavy periods that may last longer than usual. There may be spotting or bleeding between periods, pain during sexual intercourse, and painful bowel movements or urination. Endometriosis can make you feel very tired or even exhausted. You are more likely to get endometriosis if you have heavy or long periods and a short cycle, if you began your periods at an early age and if you have a close relative who has endometriosis.

'I'd always suspected that everything wasn't quite right and I started getting a lot of pain. I looked my symptoms up on the Internet and I kept coming up with endometriosis. It was the only thing that seemed to be related to bowel pain and period problems. There was at least a year when I was struggling on with pain every month, thinking that there was nothing wrong with me and I should be able to cope with it. Eventually I got referred to hospital and had a laparoscopy and I did have endometriosis.' *Gillian, 30*

Fibroids

....

Fibroids are benign tumours that grow in the womb. They are often found inside the layers of the wall of the womb, but they can also grow in the cavity of the womb or on the outer wall. Fibroids sometimes develop in the cervix, or neck of the womb. They are made up of womb muscle fibre, and can grow as big as a melon. Fibroids are only extremely rarely cancerous, but they can affect your fertility because they can make it difficult for embryos to implant, and they are also associated with miscarriage.

The majority of women who have fibroids have no symptoms and are completely unaware that they have them. Symptoms may be more or less common depending on the size of the fibroids and their position. When there are symptoms, the most common is heavy menstrual bleeding. You may also have painful periods, bloating and lower back pain. Some women experience constipation or bladder problems. Studies have found that there is a higher incidence of fibroids among black women, although the reasons for this are not clear. Women who are overweight are also more at risk.

Blocked or scarred fallopian tubes

....

If your fallopian tubes are blocked, scarred or damaged, eggs will find it difficult to get through them on their way from the ovaries to the womb. Fallopian tubes can be harmed by infection or by scar tissue if you have had any previous surgery in the pelvic area. Sometimes endometriosis can lead to tubal damage.

Pelvic inflammatory disease (PID) is a major cause of tubal problems, as it can lead to adhesions, or scar tissue, around the fallopian tubes. PID can be triggered by bacterial infection, but by far the most common cause nowadays is chlamydia, a sexually transmitted disease. Young women are particularly at risk from chlamydia, as it is estimated that around 10 per cent of sexually active young people may have the disease, which often has no symptoms at all. A woman who has chlamydia is often completely unaware that she is infected, and yet it may be seriously damaging her chances of having a child in the future.

'I'd never heard of chlamydia until I was given a leaflet saying you could have it and not know about it, so I thought I might as well have the test. It came back that I had it. I had a course of antibiotics, but about two years after that they discovered the chlamydia had never cleared up. They said it was like a gluey substance that was sticking to everything like superglue, and sticking everything down. It had got so bad that it was untreatable. It was actually sticking to my internal organs.' *Jeanette, 24*

Those most at risk of getting pelvic inflammatory disease are younger women who have multiple sexual partners, who had their first sexual experience at a young age and who have a high frequency of intercourse. It can lead to ectopic pregnancy and women who have had PID often have repeated attacks. As with chlamydia, there are often no symptoms, although some women with PID have pain in the lower abdomen, painful intercourse, fever and vaginal discharge.

Hydrosalpinx

Sometimes one of the fallopian tubes becomes completely blocked and it can swell and fill up with watery fluid. This is known as a hydrosalpinx, and is usually caused by previous infection or surgery. The fluid tends to collect at the end of the tube that is closest to the ovary. Women who have a hydrosalpinx may experience very severe pelvic pain, but it is possible to have no symptoms at all. Sometimes only one tube is affected, but it can occur in both at the same time (bilateral hydrosalpinges). If both tubes are completely blocked, the only way to get pregnant is with IVF. There is evidence that a hydrosalpinx can reduce embryo implantation rates and increase the risk of miscarriage. For this reason, women who have hydrosalpinges often have their fallopian tubes removed before starting IVF.

'The consultant said our only chance of having a baby was through IVF, but that our chances of IVF working were halved because I had bilateral hydrosalpinges. We were distraught. He said I would have to have my tubes removed. I knew they didn't work, so I thought I might as well do it right away, but there is a stigma to being sterilised at 31.'
Mikaela, 32

Physical problems with the womb or ovaries

There can be physical problems with the ovaries or the womb that make it difficult for a woman to conceive. Sometimes the outer surface of the ovaries may be scarred, usually after some kind of surgery, and this makes it difficult for follicles to develop normally. The womb is sometimes oddly shaped, and depending on how serious this is, it can lead to infertility and miscarriage.

Asherman's syndrome

The name Asherman's syndrome is given to a rare condition where scar tissue is found inside the womb. It sometimes causes the front and back walls of the womb to stick together, although in milder cases the scarring is found in just a small portion of the womb. It can be the result of a D and C (dilatation and curettage) or an ERPC (evacuation of the retained products of conception), which involve clearing the womb after a miscarriage, to remove a retained placenta or to terminate a pregnancy. Scarring can also be caused by a caesarean section or other surgery, or by infection.

The symptoms of Asherman's are usually changes to the menstrual cycle, which may become shorter or lighter than before, and sometimes stops altogether. Some women feel period pain but don't bleed. This can be a sign that although menstruation is taking place, the blood can't get out of the womb because the cervix is blocked by scar tissue.

'I had a retained placenta when I had my daughter, and I was told I had to have emergency surgery, but after the ERPC, I had more and more problems. The pain I was having was quite incredible and I didn't have a bleed. They finally referred me to a consultant and we had tests that showed my cervix was completely closed up, and I had 90–95 per cent obliteration of the uterine cavity.' *Abbi, 31*

Problems with cervical mucus

Usually cervical mucus reaches a special consistency around the time of ovulation, which makes it easier for sperm to swim through it into the womb. If this doesn't happen and the mucus is thick or very scanty, it may be impossible for the sperm to swim through it and get into the womb. This is now considered to be a very rare cause of infertility.

Immune problems

There is growing interest in reproductive immunology, which is concerned with looking at whether a woman's system may reject sperm or embryos, and prevent the implantation of a fertilised egg. Usually, your body rejects any kind of unrecognised material that starts growing inside it, but when you get pregnant, special blocking antibodies stop your immune system attacking the foetus. Some doctors believe that sometimes this blocking system fails, that the body may reject sperm or embryos, or start producing too many natural killer cells that attack growing cells in the body. Reproductive immunology is still a controversial area, and although some clinics now offer tests, others believe they are of limited use and question the validity of both the tests and the treatments offered, as most are not scientifically proven and are often expensive.

Unexplained infertility

Many couples never find out why they can't conceive, as no cause is found for their problems despite extensive tests. In some cases, it is thought that this could be down to age, despite apparently normal test results, but in most cases it is just a matter of doctors not being able to get to the root of the problem. Sixty per cent of those with unexplained infertility will conceive naturally within three years, but that still leaves many others with no idea why they can't have children.

Unexplained infertility can be a difficult diagnosis to live with, and some women find it hard not to blame themselves, wondering whether it is something they have done in the past which has caused the problem, or even something they are still doing unawares. Not knowing what you are up against can make the whole experience particularly difficult.

'I have unexplained infertility, which is not reassuring at all. All it means is that they haven't found anything with the tests they have these days. I think unexplained infertility is a bit of a cop out. You think, is it me? Is it my problem I'm not conceiving because I'm stressing out so much? Is it the food I'm eating? Is it because I'm 37?' *Lana, 37*

Secondary infertility

Women who have already been pregnant don't expect to have problems conceiving again, but in fact as many as a third of the patients at fertility clinics will have had a child, or a pregnancy, in the past. This is known as secondary infertility.

Some conditions which affect fertility can develop after a first pregnancy, such as endometriosis, hormone imbalances or sperm problems. An untreated infection after a previous delivery can leave scar tissue, or block the fallopian tubes. Women who have had a caesarean section, especially during the later stages of labour, are at slightly greater risk. Sometimes secondary infertility is simply down to age. If a couple have relatively minor fertility problems and start trying for a first child when they are fairly young, they may still manage to conceive, but if the minor problems are combined with age, it can make all the difference. In some cases, secondary infertility will remain unexplained.

It is important not to assume you cannot possibly have a fertility problem just because you've already conceived before. If you've been trying unsuccessfully for another baby for more than a year, it is worth having some basic tests carried out.

Possible causes from your male partner

Most male fertility problems involve sperm. There may be a low sperm count (not enough sperm in the semen), there may be problems with sperm motility (the sperm aren't moving properly) or with sperm morphology (the sperm may be abnormal). Having a varicocele in the testicles, which is a bit like a varicose vein, can damage sperm, as it affects the blood flow. Some sperm problems are hormonal and some may be genetic, whereas others are caused by infection, but quite often there is no obvious cause for the problem.

Sometimes there is agglutination in the semen sample, which means the sperm are stuck together in clumps and can't fertilise an egg. This is often caused by anti-sperm antibodies in the blood, which may be the result of injury or surgery.

In some cases, there are simply no sperm in the semen sample at all. This is usually due to some kind of blockage, but can also happen when a man doesn't have a tube linking his testes to his penis (the vas deferens), when the muscles that pump the sperm out aren't working properly or because no sperm are produced in the testes. It is important to remember that smoking, excess alcohol and recreational drugs can all affect sperm production, and male fertility problems can be caused by these lifestyle factors.

'My partner has poor sperm morphology. There were a very tiny percentage of normal sperm, and all the rest were not normal. I think sometimes he felt slightly guilty about it. I would have much preferred it if it had been me. That would have made it a lot easier. But it wasn't. It's nobody's fault, it's just one of those things that happen.' *Anna, 33*

Chapter seven

Fertility Tests

When women first start the process of fertility testing, all any of us really want to know is whether there is anything wrong, and whether we will be able to have a baby. Unfortunately, fertility tests don't always give the clear-cut answers we are looking for. Although they can pinpoint particular problems, the results are sometimes rather ambiguous, and you can go through a whole battery of tests and still emerge none the wiser as to why you aren't getting pregnant.

The other main problem with fertility tests is that they seem to take so long. Testing is a matter of elimination, so doctors will start with the most straightforward test and work their way through the others until they find a clue as to what may be causing problems. There are often long gaps in between tests where you are waiting for results, and then waiting for the next appointment. It can be very frustrating, especially if you are starting to worry about your age and feeling that your biological clock is ticking away, and your fertility is declining, while you wait. Paying for tests privately can sometimes speed up the process and reduce waiting time for appointments, but it can still take a while if the results prove inconclusive and you have to work your way through a number of different procedures.

'I expected that you would go straight to the doctor and they would tell you what was wrong with you. I didn't know a lot about infertility and how they go about diagnosing it. I didn't realise how long it took to get to the bottom of what the problem was.' *Rachel, 35*

Medical history

Your doctor will probably want to begin any assessment of your fertility by looking at your medical history. Your age, weight and menstrual cycle pattern may be relevant, and details of any previous surgery or sexually transmitted diseases can help form a picture of potential problem areas. Your doctor may also want to do an internal pelvic examination at this stage, and a cervical smear.

Your partner's medical history is important too, and your doctor needs to consider the two of you as a couple in order to work out where any problems could lie. Your partner should have a physical examination, as this can highlight any problems with the testicles or the tubes leading away from the testicles, which carry the sperm.

Blood tests

The first test you are likely to have is a blood test to check your hormone levels. These tests have to be carried out at the right point in your cycle. Doctors usually do a progesterone test to make sure you have ovulated, as progesterone is produced by the ovaries after an egg has been released and good progesterone levels indicate that you are ovulating normally. The progesterone test is done on day 21 of a regular 28-day cycle. If your cycle is shorter or longer, it is important to make sure that the timing is adjusted, as the results won't be accurate if the test is done at the wrong time. If you have irregular periods, it is going to be much harder to work out when you are ovulating, and you may have to have a series of blood tests to check your progesterone levels.

You should also have a test for the hormones that stimulate the ovaries to produce eggs. These are follicle-stimulating hormone (FSH) and luteinising hormone (LH), and this test is normally done on day two or three of your cycle. High levels of FSH and LH indicate that your ovarian reserve (the number and quality of eggs remaining in the ovaries) is low, and this can make it harder for you to get pregnant.

If your periods are irregular, you may have a blood test to check your prolactin levels, as high levels of this hormone can affect your menstrual cycle. If doctors think thyroid disease is a possibility you may be tested for this too, as an underactive thyroid can affect egg quality and increase the risk of infertility and miscarriage.

Your doctor may also want to make sure that you are

immune to rubella (German measles). Although German measles is not usually a serious illness, it can damage a baby during early pregnancy, and if you are not immune you will be told to avoid risking pregnancy until you have been immunised.

Sometimes your family doctor will be happy to carry out some of these basic blood tests before referring you to a specialist, whereas other doctors may prefer to refer you straight away.

Sperm tests

Sperm testing is a key part of any fertility investigation, and this is usually one of the first tests carried out along with the blood tests. The man produces a sample of semen by masturbation, which is collected in a small pot for analysis in a laboratory. The sample may have to be produced at the hospital, and most fertility clinics have special rooms for this purpose. The idea of performing to order in a back room at the clinic with a few erotic magazines for company can be deeply unappealing, and some men find the whole experience difficult. If you live near the clinic it may be possible to produce a sample at home and bring it in to the laboratory. If you do get the go-ahead to do this, you must get the sample back as quickly as you can, ideally within a couple of hours, and you shouldn't let it get too cold.

It is usually recommended that you don't have intercourse for a few days before giving a sperm sample, which leads some men to assume they will have a much higher sperm count if they abstain from sex for longer than this. In fact, although abstaining for weeks may produce a higher volume of seminal fluid, there is often a decreased percentage of live, active sperm, so this isn't advisable.

The sperm test involves a number of checks to make sure the sample is normal and full of healthy sperm. The volume of fluid is checked, and it is examined to see how quickly it liquefies, which normally happens fairly soon after it has been ejaculated. The sample is examined under a microscope to see how many sperm are present (the sperm concentration) and to make sure the sperm are swimming fast enough and going forwards rather than moving erratically or just twitching about (this is known as the motility). The sperm should not be stuck together (agglutination) as this can suggest there are antisperm antibodies present. The shape of the sperm (sperm morphology) will also be observed, as they sometimes have abnormally shaped heads or tails. The number of white blood cells may be checked, as high levels can indicate infection. Sometimes a sperm antibody test is also carried out, which checks for antibodies that can affect the way the sperm function and prevent them fertilising an egg.

Sperm counts can vary considerably, and a normally fertile man may produce a sample with a low count at certain times, so it is worth repeating the sperm test if the results do suggest there could be a problem. Sperm production is a slow process, which takes about three months, and illness, medication or excess alcohol consumption during this period may affect the count.

Chlamydia screening

Chlamydia, a sexually transmitted disease, can cause fertility problems if it is not diagnosed. Chlamydia testing is simple and usually just involves taking a urine sample or a swab. If the results are positive, you and your partner will be prescribed a course of antibiotics. As chlamydia has no symptoms it can affect your fertility without your knowledge and if it has already caused damage to your fallopian tubes, the antibiotics will not be able to reverse this.

Ultrasound scans

A relatively unobtrusive way of looking at the ovaries, ultrasound scans can show how follicles are developing and whether there are any cysts that could suggest polycystic ovaries. An ultrasound scan can also give a view of the womb itself, and it is possible to check the lining to make sure it seems to be about the right thickness for the stage of the menstrual cycle.

Unlike pregnancy scans where the ultrasound probe is used externally on the stomach, most of the scans carried out during infertility investigations are done internally (known as transvaginal ultrasound scans), as this gives a clearer view of your reproductive organs. The scan works by using sound waves that send out echoes as they bounce off your body and these are used to give a picture.

At first, a transvaginal scan may feel rather odd and undignified, but they are painless and quite straighforward. You will need to take off the clothes you are wearing on the bottom half of your body, and lie on a bed. The doctor then inserts the ultrasound probe into your vagina, and can look at your ovaries and follicles on a small screen.

'I had one of those internal ultrasound scans, and they detected polycystic ovaries straight away. I've had several scans now, and they're absolutely fine. I found the first one really informative as well, because they showed me exactly what was wrong. They pointed out the cysts on my ovaries, so I actually found it very helpful for me to understand.'
Lucy, 27

Follicle tracking

Doctors sometimes use follicle tracking to allow them to assess how well your follicles develop during a cycle, and to monitor ovulation. It may be particularly useful if you are taking a fertility drug, as this will give an indication of how effectively it is working. Follicle tracking involves a series of scans during the first half of the menstrual cycle. Follicles can be measured to see how well they are growing, as we know that when they reach a certain size the egg is usually mature and ready to burst out of the follicle.

Hysterosalpingogram

A hysterosalpingogram, known as an HSG, is a procedure that uses X-ray pictures to look at the condition of the womb and fallopian tubes. It can be carried out in an outpatient clinic and you don't need an anaesthetic. During an HSG, dye is injected into a tube, which is passed into the womb through the vagina and cervix. A series of X-rays are taken as the dye travels through the womb and tubes. The pictures will show up any blockages, kinks in the tubes, adhesions, fibroids (see Chapter 6) or any other growths. Some women find the HSG very uncomfortable, and experience considerable pain and cramping. Others don't have any problems with it at all.

'The HSG was a terrible experience. I know it varies from person to person, but I found it very uncomfortable. They got the fluid in, and they took the pictures, but it was just very painful.' *Emma, 33*

'The HSG was not as bad as they'd told me it would be. Uncomfortable, very undignified, but not actually painful.' *Corinne, 36*

Hysterosalpingo-contrast sonography

HyCoSy, or hysterosalpingo-contrast sonography, is very similar to the HSG and also allows an assessment of the condition of the tubes, but it uses ultrasound rather than X-ray. A tube is put through the cervix and a 'contrast medium' (a liquid that will show up brightly on the scan) is injected into the womb. A transvaginal ultrasound scan is used to look at the inside of the womb and rule out any fibroids or polyps. As the contrast medium flows along the fallopian tubes it will highlight any blockages or adhesions. The HyCoSy is carried out in an outpatient clinic, and usually takes half an hour at the most. Some women experience period-type pains with the HyCoSy, and are advised to take painkillers.

'I'd heard lots of awful things about the HyCoSy – that it was really uncomfortable and painful and things, and that you feel pretty awful afterwards. You get a bit worried, but actually it was not as bad as I thought. I had a bit of pain while they were doing it, but it was just like having stomach cramps, and I had cramps afterwards.' *Paula, 34*

Laparoscopy and dye

A laparoscopy and dye test is an operation that has to be carried out under general anaesthetic, although you can usually go home a few hours afterwards so it doesn't involve an overnight stay in hospital. During the test, the doctor uses a tiny telescope (laparoscope) to look at the condition of the womb and fallopian tubes.

Once you are asleep, the doctor makes a small cut just beneath your navel, and your abdomen is inflated with carbon dioxide to give a clear view. Then the laparoscope is put through the incision, and dye is injected through the tubes to make sure they are clear, or 'patent'. If there are no blockages or scarring, the dye passes through the tubes freely and spills out the ends.

The laparoscopy does not usually cause any problems, although you will probably feel some discomfort around the cut, and you may feel bloated or have a stomach ache.

There is also sometimes pain around the shoulder, which is caused by the left-over gas in the abdomen. Some women, particularly those who have never had a general anaesthetic before, find the prospect of an operation rather alarming, but a laparoscopy is a fairly standard fertility investigation. It is often suggested when there is suspected endometriosis or a history of pelvic inflammatory disease, and can give a more detailed assessment of any blockages or adhesions that have shown up on an HSG or HyCoSy.

'I've had quite a few laparoscopies and they aren't too bad. The recovery time can be up to a week and I did have shoulder pain, but it really didn't feel too bad. There's nothing to worry about. I had my appendix out this year, and that was much worse.' *Gillian, 34*

Hysteroscopy

A hysteroscopy is an examination of the womb that involves putting a small telescope (hysteroscope) through the cervix. It may be carried out when you are having a laparoscopy, or can be done separately. You will be given a local anaesthetic or some form of sedation before the hysteroscopy is carried out. The hysteroscopy gives a good view of the inside of the womb, but is usually offered only where there is a reason to suspect there may be problems. Fibroids (see Chapter 7), adhesions or any irregularities in the shape of the womb can be assessed with a hysteroscopy.

Post-coital tests

Although post-coital tests were once offered routinely to women who weren't getting pregnant, they are rarely carried out now. The test involves having sex at home with your partner and then going to the clinic for an internal examination some hours later. A sample of cervical mucus is taken and examined under a micro-scope to see how well the sperm are surviving. The test should be carried out around the time of ovulation when the cervical mucus is copious and watery, allowing sperm to move freely. Immediately after ovulation, the cervical mucus becomes thick and sticky and it is hard for sperm to get through it, and a test carried out at the wrong time can produce a false negative, wrongly suggesting that there may be problems.

'It was the most embarrassing test of all. The first thing the doctor asked me was how many hours it was since we'd had sex. I just wanted to curl up and disappear. He had a medical student with him, so he was explaining everything as he did it, which made it all a million times worse. They sat there peering at my husband's sperm swimming about, and discussing what they looked like, and what they should look like, but I wasn't even interested in the result – all I could think of was how much I wanted to get out of there.'
Carol, 45

Reproductive immunology

Still fairly new, reproductive immunology is a rather controversial area of fertility testing and treatment. It is based around the idea that the female immune system may react against sperm and embryos, stopping fertilisation and implantation or causing miscarriage.

It may be suggested that you should have tests to check whether your immune system could be preventing you getting pregnant or maintaining a pregnancy. Usually this will mean having blood tests, but you may be offered other tests, such as an endometrial biopsy where a small piece of the womb lining is taken out for further testing, and you may then be offered treatment. The test results may suggest that you have raised antibodies, or higher than normal levels of the natural killer (NK) cells that we all carry in our bodies.

There are only a few clinics offering these tests, as many doctors consider them to be of limited value. They say, for example, that testing levels of NK cells in the blood is of little use as they are totally different to the NK cells that are found in the womb. If you've had recurrent miscarriages, or a number of unsuccessful IVF attempts, you may consider investigating this area, but it is important to remember that these tests and treatments are still in their infancy and are not scientifically proven.

Chapter eight

Fertility Treatment

When we talk about fertility treatment, it is usually IVF and other assisted conception techniques that spring to mind, but there may be much simpler solutions for some women who are having difficulty getting pregnant. Your individual situation and the nature of your fertility problem will determine the type of treatment that is appropriate.

Drug treatments

Many women are offered some kind of fertility drug as a first treatment, which can boost your fertility if you have ovulation problems.

Clomifene citrate and tamoxifen

Clomifene citrate is probably the most commonly prescribed drug, along with tamoxifen. These drugs are used to stimulate the ovaries. Clomifene citrate can help women who don't usually ovulate to produce eggs, and can regulate your cycle if you aren't ovulating every month.

It may also be given to women who have unexplained infertility. Although the drug undoubtedly helps many women to conceive, it is sometimes prescribed in a rather ad hoc fashion to anyone who is trying to get pregnant unsuccessfully, when there may be other fertility problems that have not been identified.

Clomifene citrate is given in the form of tablets, which are taken for five days each month early in the menstrual cycle. Women usually start with a dose of 50mg, which may be increased if you aren't responding to the drug. It is not advisable to take clomifene citrate for more than six months at a time, as there are questions about long-term use of the drug and possible links to ovarian cancer.

When you are taking clomifene citrate, you should be monitored to check whether you are ovulating. Some women are given the drug without any checks or monitors, and so have no idea whether it is working, whereas others may be offered just blood tests. It is good practice to monitor the use of clomifene citrate or tamoxifen with ultrasound scans in at least the first cycle, as this allows doctors to see how your ovaries are responding. It can also alert them if there is a risk of a multiple pregnancy, as the drugs may stimulate the ovaries to produce not just one but a number of viable eggs.

'They put me straight on clomifene. They didn't check whether ovulation was a problem. They weren't tracking me at all. I was on these strong drugs with no supervision. I had no appointment to go back. It was a situation of take this and go away for six months even though the drug is probably going to do nothing for you.' *Nicol, 33*

Some women take clomifene citrate and tamoxifen without any problems, but others have unpleasant side effects. These are usually described in literature about the drugs as menopausal symptoms such as headaches and hot flushes. In fact, what most women find difficult to cope with is the way the drug affects their moods.

'The first time I took clomifene I had really bad mood swings and was depressed. I didn't get many physical side effects; it was more emotional and mental. I did take it first thing in the morning, but now I take it at night, so hopefully I sleep through the worst of it. I've just had it this month and I've had pains and hot flushes. It's the first time it has affected me like that.' *Lisa, 32*

Metformin

Women with polycystic ovary syndrome may be offered metformin, either instead of or along with clomifene citrate. Metformin was developed to treat age-related diabetes by lowering blood-sugar levels and reducing high insulin levels. Women who have PCOS (see Chapter 6) produce high levels of insulin. Metformin can help by making the body more sensitive to insulin, which means less is produced. However, it is not licensed for use for fertility problems, as it was not originally intended for this purpose.

Metformin is most commonly prescribed for women who have PCOS who are also overweight, and for those who haven't responded to clomifene citrate or tamoxifen. Combining metformin with these drugs increases the chances of ovulation. Metformin works better for women who are overweight, although it is no substitute for weight loss. The drug can have side effects such as nausea, vomiting and diarrhoea.

> 'Just for a few weeks I had some bad side effects. I had diarrhoea, and was a little bit sick, but once that wore off I've not had anything since. I think some women just don't get over the side effects of metformin and simply aren't able to take it, but I got used to it relatively quickly.' *Lucy, 27*

Gonadotrophin hormone treatment

Hormone treatment using gonadotrophins is the next level of drug treatment for women with ovulatory problems. Follicle-stimulating hormone (FSH) and luteinising hormone (LH) are gonadotrophins, which are produced naturally in our bodies, and are a vital part of our reproductive cycle. The drugs using these hormones may contain just FSH alone, or FSH and LH, and are given by injection. When you are taking these drugs it is essential that you are properly monitored using ultrasound, as there is a risk of multiple births. It is also possible that the ovaries can be overstimulated, leading to ovarian hyperstimulation syndrome (OHSS), which can pose serious health problems.

Bromocriptine, cabergoline and dopamine agonists

These drugs may be prescribed for women who have a disorder of the pituitary gland called hyperprolactinaemia, which causes them to produce too much prolactin. This condition can lead to irregular periods, and thus infertility. These drugs can have side effects such as nausea, sickness, headaches and dizziness.

Laparoscopic ovarian drilling

Laparoscopic ovarian drilling is sometimes offered to women with polycystic ovaries, particularly those who have not responded to clomifene citrate. It involves a general anaesthetic and a laparoscopy. A tiny telescope (a laparoscope) is inserted through a small incision into the abdomen, and heat is used to burn small holes on the surface of the ovaries. This process seems to help trigger ovulation in some women.

'They go in through the belly button and they make holes all over the ovaries. It was only day surgery, and I was home in the evening. It was a little bit tender, but painless. The only discomfort you have is in your shoulder from the build up of gas, but it does go very quickly if you lie flat for a couple of hours.' *Sarah, 34*

Treatment for problems with fallopian tubes

There are a number of procedures that may be offered to patients who have blocked or damaged fallopian tubes to try to clear the tubes so that eggs can pass freely along them and pregnancy can occur. One of the simplest ways to try to unblock the tubes involves using a fine catheter, which is inserted through the cervix. A narrow wire is pushed through the catheter to try to clear the blockage away. The process is often successful, but does carry a risk of damaging or perforating the tube, and some women find it painful. Sometimes doctors try to clear blockages in the tubes by inserting a small balloon into the tubes and inflating it.

Tubal surgery

It may be possible to remove blockages in the tubes and scar tissue by surgery. Women who have blocked tubes are now generally offered IVF rather than surgery, as this by-passes the fallopian tubes, and has a higher chance of producing a pregnancy. If surgery is offered, it should be done laparoscopically, and the chances of success will depend on the nature and severity of the problem. Sometimes a blocked portion of tube will be cut out and the ends joined together, and scar tissue, which can glue up the reproductive organs by covering them like sticky cobwebs, can be removed.

Tubal surgery is only generally considered when both tubes are blocked. Although it will probably take longer to get pregnant with just one open tube, there is a risk that attempting to repair the blocked tube could leave scarring that might damage the clear tube. There is an increased risk of ectopic pregnancy after tubal surgery.

Uterine surgery

Some women will be offered surgery to remove fibroids or scar tissue in the womb. Many of these operations on the womb are now done using keyhole surgery where possible, rather than open surgery.

Intrauterine insemination (IUI)

IUI, or intrauterine insemination, may be offered to couples with unexplained infertility, for women with mild endometriosis or polycystic ovary syndrome and for minor male factor sperm problems. IUI is often suggested as a precursor to IVF, as it is less invasive and less expensive.

During an IUI treatment cycle, the man's sperm is placed inside his partner's womb to increase the chances of pregnancy. IUI is sometimes carried out without using any fertility drugs, in what is called an unstimulated cycle. Alternatively, drugs may be used to induce ovulation in a stimulated cycle, but this increases the risk of a multiple birth.

During an IUI cycle, the follicles that are developing in the ovaries are regularly monitored with ultrasound to check on their progress, and you may be asked to use an ovulation prediction kit too. When the time is right, you go to the clinic where your partner is asked to produce a sperm sample. The sample is 'washed', which ensures only good-quality sperm are used for the insemination. They are put right into the womb in a thin catheter, which is passed through the cervix.

Usually, you will have the sperm put into the womb only once during each cycle. Some clinics do offer two inseminations, but there is no evidence that this improves the chances of a successful outcome. If you are having IUI, do check that your clinic is open at weekends and bank holidays. Otherwise, if you ovulate at the wrong time, the treatment won't be able to go ahead.

> 'It was fairly nightmarish. We'd go through it all, and then if I ovulated at the weekend or on a bank holiday, that was that. They couldn't do the treatment. I found it so stressful. We never knew if we would have the treatment or not.' *Lulu, 39*

You may be offered up to six cycles of IUI, although few couples actually seem to get through that many, often preferring to move on to IVF if the IUI is unsuccessful. The success rates for an individual cycle of IUI are not high, at around 12 per cent, but the chances of getting pregnant are increased in stimulated cycles. IUI is often regarded as much 'easier' than IVF from the patient's perspective, but the emotional trauma of unsuccessful treatment cycles is the same, and some women find it just as hard to deal with.

> 'I did IUI for six months. There was always a risk that you would either overdo it or under-do it, so one month the cycle would be cancelled because I didn't have any follicles, and the next month it would be cancelled because there were too many, because if there were more than three they wouldn't inseminate. It was stressful. You just felt like you never knew where you were.' *Naomi, 39*

IVF

One of the most established forms of assisted reproduction, IVF has been used for about 30 years. IVF stands for 'in-vitro fertilisation', and it involves eggs being taken out of the woman's body and fertilised with her partner's sperm in a laboratory, before being returned to the womb as embryos. Most couples don't imagine they will ever get as far down the line of treatment as IVF, and it can be a daunting prospect.

There is a general assumption, probably partly because we have all read so much about miracle test-tube babies, that IVF will inevitably work. In fact, even now with much improved success rates, an individual IVF cycle is more likely to fail than it is to succeed. That can be hard to accept when you are investing so much emotion, time and often money too, in your first treatment cycle.

'You go into it quite naively really. You hear about IVF in the media, and you think you do IVF and get a baby at the end. Thinking back we were so unrealistic. We went into the first one really excited and hopeful, thinking that now we were going to get our baby. It was only when the first one failed that we realised actually it doesn't work like that.' *Mary, 38*

Before you start an IVF cycle, you may be asked to take a number of tests for HIV, hepatitis B and hepatitis C. These tests are necessary to rule out the risk of passing these infections on to other people or to a baby. If you do test positive, the clinic will have to take a decision as to whether they will proceed with the treatment.

IVF can be carried out in a normal cycle, without any

drugs being used. This is known as natural-cycle IVF. It is cheaper, and does not run the risk of over-stimulating the ovaries, but it is much less likely to be successful. The vast majority of IVF treatment involves the use of drugs to stimulate the ovaries so that they produce a number of eggs, giving more chance that some will fertilise and develop. Some doctors are now looking at the possibility of milder stimulation using fewer drugs, which is known as 'soft IVF'.

Your clinic will normally arrange some kind of introduction to the IVF process. This may be a chat with a doctor or nurse who will explain it to you as a couple, or it may be a much larger affair. It is important to understand as much as you can about what is going to happen during the cycle, as this will make the process easier.

You will usually begin your IVF treatment with a period of 'down-regulation' where you are given drugs that switch off your own hormonal cycle and stop the ovaries producing eggs. This allows the medical team to have closer control over your ovaries. The down-regulation drugs are generally taken either as a nasal spray or an injection. Some women experience menopausal symptoms during down-regulation, which can be unpleasant, ranging from hot flushes to headaches. Sometimes a shorter treatment plan may be used where the down-regulation drugs are not taken so early on.

Once the body's natural cycle has been switched off, drugs are used to stimulate the ovaries so that they will produce a number of eggs – a process known as superovulation. Gonadotrophins (FSH and LH) are used for this purpose. Some drugs have just FSH, some have LH and FSH. Originally the drugs used for superovulation were made using the purified urine of menopausal women, which is why you may have heard stories about lorry-loads of urine being collected from convents where there were concentrations of menopausal women all excreting FSH. Now, many of the drugs are made in the laboratory without the need to extract the hormones from human urine. They are known as recombinant drugs, and are, rather bizarrely, sometimes produced using Chinese hamster ovaries. There are large differences in the cost of the different types of drugs used for superovulation, but little evidence to suggest that the more expensive drugs are any more effective. There are not usually too many unpleasant side effects with the drugs, although many women do feel bloated as their ovaries respond, and it is common to feel very emotional at this time.

'When the drugs start kicking in, you do start getting a little bit emotional. I think my husband saw me becoming more and more stressed. I felt I was holding things together pretty well, but I think he felt that I wasn't a lot of the time. I did let things affect me a lot more. It was only looking back on it that I realised how weird I must have been at that time, really obsessing about things.' *Heather, 48*

One of the things many couples find most alarming about starting IVF is the fact that the drugs are given by injection, which they are expected to do themselves at home. Some women get their partners to do it, and find it helps them to feel involved, others prefer to do it themselves. The clinic will give help, advice and practice at injecting before they send you off home with a pack of syringes and drugs, and self-injecting kits are now available which make it much easier. Most couples find they cope with it all surprisingly well, but it is often a source of worry.

'It was kind of terrifying. My husband is a bit phobic about needles, but there was no way I could do it myself. The nurse did the very first injection. He watched her do it and he said he thought he could do that. We got into a kind of routine. I'd prepare it and load up the syringe and he would do it. I think it brought us closer together, that he would do it for me and that I trusted him to do it.' *Gillian, 30*

Sometimes it is the day-to-day practicalities of the injections that can be the most difficult thing to deal with.

'I didn't actually mind the injecting. You have to do it at a particular time of day, and I was never sure I was going to be at exactly the right place. I was injecting in my office and keeping all sorts of injection equipment under the desk and not being able to figure out how to get the syringes home and into my sharps box. I was injecting in the library, injecting on a railway … None of it really did me any harm, but it was stressful.' *Naomi, 39*

Once you have got underway with the injections, you will have to go back to the clinic for monitoring. The medical team use ultrasound to check the follicles and when they have reached the right size, and the womb lining is thick enough, it is time to ripen them. This is done with an injection of a hormone that helps eggs mature. Often this injection has to be given late at night, and the timing is very important.

The next stage is egg collection. You both go back to the clinic, where the male partner is asked to give a sperm sample. Some men find there is a lot of pressure to perform, which can make them anxious about doing this, and it is may be possible to freeze sperm in advance if you are worried that this could be a problem. The woman is then heavily sedated, or sometimes completely knocked out with a general anaesthetic, so that the eggs can be collected. Ultrasound is used to identify the follicles and then a thin needle is inserted into them through the vagina, and the fluid is sucked out of each follicle. Not all follicles contain eggs, but if there is one inside, it will come out in the fluid.

'I had been quite anxious about the egg retrieval. I thought it would be very painful. I hadn't actually realised until about a week before that they took the eggs out through the vaginal wall. In the end I had a general anaesthetic so it was really that that I was recovering from. It was pretty gruelling.'
Naomi, 39

The embryologist mixes the eggs and sperm together in a dish, and puts them in an incubator. The sperm won't usually fertilise every egg, but the eggs that have been fertilised should start dividing. After two or three days, one or two embryos can be transferred to the womb, or they may be left for longer to develop into blasto-cysts, which are more mature embryos. Not all embryos will survive long enough in the laboratory to become blastocysts, but those that do have a higher chance of implanting.

Embryo transfer is carried out when the embryo, or embryos, are ready to be replaced and is usually a straight-forward procedure that doesn't involve any anaesthetic. The embryo is put into a thin catheter and passed into the womb through the cervix. Ultrasound is used to make sure it has gone into the right place, and then you are usually asked to lie still for a little while before being allowed home. After embryo transfer, you may be given progesterone supplements to help the embryo implant in the womb.

If you have produced a good number of embryos, those you are not having replaced can be frozen. Clinics usually only freeze good-quality embryos, and not all of them will survive the freezing and thawing process.

The two weeks that follow embryo transfer, known as the 'two-week wait' is often described as the most diffi-cult part of IVF treatment. Up until this point, you have been busily moving towards the goal of embryo transfer. Once this is done, there is nothing more you can do except wait.

'The two-week wait was horrendous. That's definitely the worst part. One day I'd be convinced I had tiny symptoms, and the next day I was convinced I had my period and it was all over. I wasn't sure whether to go back to work or not, but I thought if I didn't I was going to go insane. I'm glad I did because there would have been too much time to think about it. At least I had a bit of distraction at work.'
Gillian, 30

Most clinics like you to go back at the end of the two-week waiting period for a blood test to see whether you are pregnant or not. Usually, the result will be a clear positive or negative, but sometimes it can be ambiguous. Although the pregnancy hormone levels are raised, they are not as high as they should be, and there is a risk that the pregnancy will not survive. This can be a particularly difficult outcome. You cannot celebrate a pregnancy at last, neither can you go off and try to forget about it for a while. Some women who begin with a low positive go on to have perfectly successful pregnancies, for others the pregnancy is eventually lost after a period of heartache.

Assisted hatching

The process of assisted hatching is sometimes used to try to increase the chances of success with IVF, often for older women or those who have had repeatedly unsuccessful attempts. It involves thinning the outer layer of the embryo or making a small hole in it before transferring it into the womb. The idea is that this may help the embryo implant, but there is no clear evidence that it makes a difference to the outcome.

Frozen embryo transfer

If you've had spare embryos frozen, you can have them transferred later in a separate treatment cycle. The frozen embryos are thawed and can be replaced in a natural cycle if you ovulate normally. If you have an irregular cycle, or have ovulation problems, your clinic may suggest taking some fertility drugs when you are going to transfer the embryos.

Going through a frozen embryo cycle is less invasive

than a full IVF cycle, and although you will need to be closely monitored to make sure the embryos are put into the womb at the optimum moment in the cycle, it is generally far less intrusive. The embryo transfer is done in the same way as during a normal IVF cycle, and is then followed by the same two-week wait.

'The frozen cycle was fantastic. I felt completely fine. There was none of the pain of egg collection, none of the worry. In fact, I felt a bit of a fraud.' *Elaine, 39*

'It was easier because I wasn't having the injections and things, but it wasn't any easier when it didn't work. That was just the same, if not worse.' *Sheona, 44*

ICSI

ICSI, or Intra-cytoplasmic sperm injection, is a type of IVF that is recommended for men with low sperm counts. ICSI is now carried out widely, despite being a relatively new process. Most of an ICSI cycle is exactly the same as IVF, but sperm is injected into the egg rather than being left to fertilise it naturally. This increases the chances of successful fertilisation, and ICSI may be offered if there have been problems with this in a previous IVF cycle. For more severe male fertility problems where there are no sperm in the semen at all, it may be possible to first remove some sperm from the testicles surgically and then carry out ICSI.

GIFT/ZIFT

Gamete intra-fallopian transfer (GIFT) and zygote intra-fallopian transfer (ZIFT) are variations of IVF, neither of which are carried out very often now. During a GIFT cycle, the eggs are collected from the woman's ovaries, but instead of being fertilised in a laboratory, they are returned to the fallopian tube along with the partner's sperm. ZIFT involves embryos being transferred to the fallopian tubes rather than the womb after the eggs have been fertilised in the laboratory.

IVM

IVM, or in-vitro maturation, is a new process pioneered in Denmark that involves taking immature eggs from the ovaries and maturing them in the laboratory before mixing them with sperm. This technique is less expensive than IVF and doesn't involve the use of such strong fertility drugs, which would be very welcome for many patients. Research in the field is ongoing, and IVM is not yet widely available.

PGD

PGD, or pre-implantation genetic diagnosis, is used to help couples who risk passing on certain inherited conditions to their children. The couple go through a normal IVF cycle, but the embryos are left to develop in the laboratory until they have divided into eight cells. An embryologist will then extract one or two cells from the embryo in order to test them for the inherited condition. Any embryos that are affected are not used, but those that are clear can be implanted or frozen for future use. PGD can help couples who risk passing on a wide range of conditions such as cystic fibrosis, muscular dystrophy, haemophilia or sickle-cell anaemia.

PGS

PGS, or pre-implantation genetic screening, is similar to PGD, as cells are taken from the embryo in the same way, but PGS checks for any chromosomal problems in the embryos that might cause miscarriage or abnormality. PGS may be offered to women who are older or to any others who are more at risk of chromosomal problems.

Ovarian hyperstimulation syndrome

Ovarian hyperstimulation syndrome (OHSS), is a fairly rare, but potentially dangerous, side effect of ovulation induction. The ovaries can become enlarged, and fluid may start to build up in the abdomen and around the lungs. During IVF monitoring, it should be apparent if you are at risk of developing OHSS, and doctors can take action to prevent you getting ill. If you are producing far too many follicles and your oestrogen levels are very high, the cycle may be halted. Usually it can be treated by bed rest and drinking lots of fluids.

The symptoms of OHSS include stomach ache, bloating, nausea and vomiting, breathing difficulties and faintness. If the condition develops, you would have to be admitted to hospital, as OHSS can be very serious, leading to thrombosis, heart attack, stroke or, in extreme cases, death. OHSS is more common among younger women and those who have polycystic ovarian syndrome.

'Nobody had really told me about the problems with hyper-stimulation. They got 26 eggs and they were worried because my oestrogen levels were quite high. For a day or so I felt fine and then I kept being sick and I felt swollen. It just got progressively worse. My weight went up half a stone per day for about four days. They put a drain on my stomach because my abdomen was full of fluid, around my kidneys and liver. My legs filled up with water. We were both very frightened.' *Elaine, 39*

Immunological problems

Women who have had recurrent miscarriages are often offered tests to check whether they are producing too many antibodies, which may cause problems. Certain antibodies cause the blood to clot more easily, and this may lead to problems if the clots are in the blood vessels of the placenta. Around 15 per cent of women who have had repeated miscarriages have high levels of these antibodies, and they are usually offered low doses of either aspirin or heparin, or both, before conception and/or during early pregnancy.

Some doctors now believe that high levels of other antibodies could be a cause of infertility. They may offer testing and treatment for immunological problems to patients with fertility problems, in case raised antibodies could be preventing implantation or attacking an embryo. There are many different types of antibodies, and many types of tests, including one to look at levels of natural killer (NK) cells. There is still much scepticism about the true value of such tests, which are often expensive.

If testing suggests you may have immunological problems, there are a variety of treatments on offer, ranging from simple doses of aspirin or heparin to more complex therapies. You may be offered steroids, rheumatoid arthritis drugs or intravenous immunoglobulin G treatment (IVIg). It is important to be aware that these treatments are not licensed for use in reproductive medicine, that they are not scientifically proven, and that they may have side effects.

Such treatment can be very costly, and you will want to think carefully before signing up for it. For those who have had repeatedly unsuccessful IVF attempts, or recurrent miscarriages, it may seem worth trying, but you should discuss it carefully with your consultant first and make sure you are quite clear why you are being offered this treatment, what exactly it is meant to do, and that you are aware of any potential risks or side effects. There is no doubt that more research needs to be done in this area before such treatments can be widely recommended. IVIg infusion treatment is usually given before and after egg collection, but it may also be offered to prevent miscarriage after a positive pregnancy test, although again there is no scientific proof that it can do this.

'My husband presented me with a pile of print-outs all saying this is unproven medicine, it is far too expensive and he said he thought it was a bit of a rip-off. But I'd had a positive pregnancy test, and I said I couldn't risk not doing it. The process was strange, to be with six or seven women for hours on end, all attached to drips. I only had one lot of IVIg and then when I went for my scan the following week there was absolutely nothing there when they scanned me.'
Debbie, 44

The cost of treatment

One real problem for many couples is the cost of fertility treatment. Although some may get limited access to funded treatment, the majority of couples do end up having to pay themselves. For affluent professionals, this may not pose huge problems, but for anyone who doesn't have much spare cash, it can be a real hurdle, making treatment effectively inaccessible.

'The consultant said, "You can decide what sort of treatment you want, these are the costs." It was like, here's the sweet shop, if you have some money, you can have what you like. It's basically what you can pay for, and we can't afford any of them. You could borrow fifteen thousand, twenty thousand, and that still might not be enough. All that, and then you don't succeed, or you get pregnant and then you have a miscarriage.' *Ellie, 44*

The risk of a multiple birth

When you take any kind of fertility-boosting drug, from clomifene to the more powerful drugs used in IVF, there is a risk of multiple pregnancy. The idea of twins, or even triplets, may seem wonderful to a woman who has spent some time trying to conceive – an instant family in one go. However, women are not designed to carry more than one baby and the natural incidence of multiple pregnancies is surprisingly low, with just 1–2 per cent of natural conceptions being twin pregnancies. The main problem with multiple pregnancies is that the babies are often born prematurely, and prematurity carries many risks. Multiple births are also more risky for mothers, who are more likely to get pre-eclampsia. Women who are going through IVF are advised to think carefully before having more than one embryo replaced in a cycle.

When fertility treatment doesn't work

When a fertility treatment you may have spent years planning and saving for doesn't work, it is devastating. The success rates for all forms of assisted conception are relatively low, and it is only when we look at cumulative success rates over two or three cycles that the picture begins to improve. One treatment cycle failing doesn't mean that treatment won't work for you eventually, but it can be hard to summon the courage to try again. Some couples are eager to throw themselves back into treatment as soon as they can, but others may benefit from some counselling and a break before they consider it again, or may want to move on to other routes to parenthood, or to coming to terms with childlessness.

'It didn't work. That was just terrible. We didn't know where to turn to. You are told over the phone and there's no follow up afterwards. I just went down into the depths of despair.' *Emma, 38*

Chapter nine

Complementary Therapies for Fertility

Although there is anecdotal evidence that complementary therapies can help women overcome fertility problems, and many men are turning to alternative treatments to try to boost low sperm counts, there is little clear scientific evidence to back this up. Today, some doctors do recommend that their patients consider complementary therapy, if only to help them feel more calm and in control. Others are deeply sceptical about any kind of alternative treatments, and worry that women may end up wasting time and money when there is no proof that these therapies have any real effect on fertility.

Despite these doubts, it is indisputable that many women find complementary therapies help them relax, and may also enable them to regain some of the control they often feel they lose when they are trying unsuccessfully to conceive. Complementary therapies are not for everyone, and some women feel happier sticking to conventional medicine.

If you go into complementary therapy looking for

miracle cures, you may be disappointed, but if you are trying to help yourself feel more relaxed, improve your sense of well-being, and perhaps even just to spend some time talking about how you feel, you may find alternative treatments very beneficial.

'I attacked complementary therapies with that sense of desperation that they'd better get me pregnant. It was very goal focused. I think, looking back, I should have done it more for relaxation. I did find all of it incredibly relaxing, but at the time it was hard when another period came round not to think, "Oh well, that didn't work." I had this mindset of looking for solutions and not really accepting that some-times there aren't any.' *Isla, 35*

Many women end up trying a variety of complementary therapies, and if you opted to go for every remedy or treat-ment that claimed to be successful at treating infertility, you could spend a very large fortune. If you have found something that is making you feel better, and which you can afford, that's never going to be a bad thing, but it is important not to get swept along into thinking that you won't get pregnant if you can't pay for lots of extra complementary treatment.

'I feel as though I've spent the same amount on comple-mentary therapies as I have on IVF, but in my mind I know I want to do that. I don't want to have missed out. If it makes me feel better and stronger, then I'll do it. I don't want to get to 45 and look back and wish I'd spent more on comple-mentary therapies.' *Lana, 37*

Complementary therapies used to boost your fertility when you are trying to get pregnant may not be recommended once you are pregnant. You should consult your therapist before continuing with any treatment if you discover you are expecting.

Acupuncture

The popular therapy acupuncture is often recommended for infertility, and is believed to be particularly helpful if there are problems related to the menstrual cycle and ovulation. Acupuncture has also been used for endometriosis and for improving the quality and quantity of sperm. There have been a number of trials that suggest acupuncture may offer real benefits to couples who are experiencing fertility problems, and one study found it could boost the chances of a successful outcome if used during IVF treatment.

Acupuncture has been practised in China for thousands of years, and is based on the idea that our body's life force, qi (pronounced chee), runs through invisible pathways or meridians under the skin. If there are blockages in these pathways, the qi cannot run freely and this is when our bodies become unbalanced and we are unwell. Acupuncture can help restore harmony by removing the blockages and helping our energy to flow again. There are more than 300 special points on the pathways around our bodies where thin needles can be inserted to clear the meridians.

'I spent quite a lot of money on things like acupuncture. I talked to nutritionists, and was brewing up Chinese herbs, but the only thing I feel really made a difference was acupuncture. I could feel a physical change. I could feel my ovaries responding. If I had a cold when I went, I could definitely feel the benefit without a doubt.' *Helena, 34*

Traditional Chinese medicine

In traditional Chinese medicine, Chinese herbs may be used, as well as acupuncture. It is based on the ancient system used in China, which classifies herbs according to their taste and the way they affect the organs and the meridians, or pathways, in the body. Some of the plants are toxic if taken in large doses, and can cause problems if combined with other herbs, so it is vital that you see a qualified practitioner before using these remedies.

Herbal medicine

Herbal medicine uses plants to treat illness and restore health. Herbs have been used in this way for centuries, and many conventional medicines still use chemicals derived from herbs. Herbalists use the entire plant to make their remedies rather than extracting the active chemical compounds from plants. Many herbal remedies are widely available, but you should see a qualified medical herbalist rather than self-prescribing something that you feel might help your situation.

'I see a herbalist who is very successful. She has got two of my friends pregnant. I take a liquid that you dilute and take in water three times a day – I've no idea what it is, and I am not sure whether it does any good, but it certainly isn't doing any harm.' *Debbie, 29*

There are some herbal remedies that are often prescribed to help with female fertility problems:

Chasteberry (*Vitex agnus-castus*) is derived from the berries of the chaste tree. It is one of the most common herbal remedies for female fertility problems, and is said to boost fertility and regulate the body's hormonal balance. It is also sometimes taken by women with high FSH levels, as it is claimed that this remedy can help bring down FSH levels.

'I took agnus castus and I do think that was a great remedy. I used to have quite painful periods that were getting shorter, and agnus castus regulated my cycle. It made my periods less painful and alleviated the symptoms I used to get pre-menstrually. People would need to check that it was right for them, but I did find it really useful. I actually got pregnant shortly after starting to take it but I lost the baby.' *Isla, 35*

Dong quai (*Angelica sinensis*) is used in traditional Chinese medicine to help with female reproductive problems. It is believed to be useful for irregular and absent periods. It should be taken only under supervision of a qualified herbalist, as in large doses it can cause changes to the menstrual flow.

False unicorn root (*Chamaelirium luteum*) was used by Native Americans to help with female reproductive problems. It is used to improve fertility where there are problems with follicles, to balance hormones and menstrual irregularities and to prevent miscarriage.

Hypnotherapy

It is sometimes suggested that a woman's subconscious can prevent her from getting pregnant. She may have hidden fears and anxieties, or problems with self-esteem. The idea of hypnotherapy is that it allows you to make contact with your subconscious mind. You are not sent to sleep, and you don't actually lose consciousness when you are hypnotised, but you are in a deeply relaxed state.

'Hypnotherapy was fantastic. I don't know if it helped me get pregnant, but I went there because my acupuncturist asked if I'd ever thought there might be something underlying that wasn't a conscious thing. I must have been to the hypnotherapist for about six months and it came up that there was something I had never been verbal about which might be stopping me from allowing myself to get pregnant.'
Alison, 38

Reflexology

In the ancient technique of reflexology parts of the body, most usually the feet, are massaged in order to help solve problems in other parts of the body. It is believed that massaging certain points, or reflex areas, which are related to specific organs, can alleviate pain or other symptoms and can help a variety of medical conditions. Reflexology is thought to be helpful for menstrual problems, and most people who have a session find it very relaxing.

'I did a course of five sessions of reflexology. The first couple of times I was amazed at how you could feel it in your body when somebody was pushing a certain area on your foot. I think towards the end I didn't feel it was doing anything. I just came away without feeling physically any different, apart perhaps from my feet feeling nice. I don't know whether I should have kept it on, but at that time it was just more expense.' *Sandra, 41*

Homeopathy

The practice of homeopathy takes a holistic approach, looking at the person as a whole rather than concentrating on individual symptoms, because it is believed that illness is related to disharmony in the body. It is based on the theory that 'like cures like', and so it uses tiny doses of substances which can produce symptoms of an illness in order to cure the illness itself. It uses medicines from plant, mineral and animal sources, which are diluted and made into tablets. It is believed that the more dilute the remedy is the more potent it becomes, as any impurities are lost. Homeopathic remedies may also be used in ointments, powders or solutions.

'Homeopathy was fantastic. The approach my homeopath took was to sit and talk about how I felt and then she would try and work out the emotional link to the physical symptoms. For me, it was just a chance to say to somebody how awful I felt about not having children. It was the first time I really recognised it. With a lot of alternative therapies there is a counselling element, and I think it was the first time I really did open up.' *Isla, 35*

Reiki

A relatively new healing technique, reiki was developed in Japan about 100 years ago. The Japanese word 'reiki' means 'universal life energy', and practitioners have to be initiated, or attuned, into this life energy by a reiki master. This then allows them to act as channels and pass the energy on to others.

During a session of reiki, you lie down while the reiki practitioner places his or her hands in a sequence of positions over your body. The process takes about an hour and it is claimed it can remove toxins and energy blocks from the body as well as passing on the life energy. It claims to be able to help with physical, mental and emotional problems, and to help you feel more relaxed and peaceful.

'A friend of mine is a reiki practitioner and before I got married she did a session. She told me that she had felt a lot of energy around my ovaries. To be quite honest I thought it was just a bit of mumbo jumbo, only to find that she had actually picked something up. That gives me confidence to go back for reiki. I just find it is extremely relaxing, and it puts you in the right frame of mind.' *Monica, 41*

Aromatherapy

The practice of aromatherapy uses concentrated essential oils derived from plants. Like herbs, plant essences have been used for their healing properties for centuries. In aromatherapy, the essential oils are added to a base oil to dilute them, and massaged into the skin. Some essential oils should not be used during pregnancy.

Aromatherapy is particularly good at relieving stress, and can improve circulation. It can be a good way of making some time for yourself in a relaxing way, and may help you feel better.

Yoga

Although yoga is not really a complementary therapy, it can help you relax, and some believe it can affect your fertility. It is claimed that yoga can strengthen your reproductive system, improve your circulation and increase blood flow to the pelvis, rebalance your hormones and even stimulate your ovaries.

'I told the teacher about my problems and one lesson she focused purely on postures to help the reproductive system. I was able to take that away and do the asanas that stimulated the ovaries at home. I've been to yoga for years, so it was just a natural progression for me.' *Angela, 32*

Holistic therapy centres

Many holistic therapy centres specialising in infertility are now springing up, offering different combinations of complementary therapies and treatments. Some also advise on diet, exercise and general health for couples who are trying to conceive, and may offer a variety of supplements, tinctures and compounds that claim to boost your fertility. These centres and their products are often expensive, which is fine if you feel you have the money and would like to spend it this way. Those who can't afford the sometimes exorbitant prices may feel this will decrease their chances of getting pregnant. In fact, much of what these centres do is aimed at making you feel more relaxed and receptive to pregnancy while improving your general health, and you may be able to do this far more cheaply yourself by making changes to your diet and lifestyle.

'You send a bit of your hair away for analysis, and they say what vitamins and minerals you are short of. At one point, we were taking 21 tablets a day of different vitamins and minerals. We spent so much money, but you get to a stage where you are so desperate that you will try anything. Occasionally I do feel bitter about all the money we spent and all the time we wasted, but at least I can look back and think we tried everything.' *Mary, 38*

With any kind of complementary therapy or alternative treatment centre, the absolutely crucial thing is to make sure you are seeing a practitioner who is registered with the appropriate professional body for his or her activity. It is also important to find somebody you feel comfortable with, as many women feel that they gain a lot of therapeutic benefit from the counselling role that complementary therapists can fill. Just taking some time out for yourself, to contemplate how you are feeling, and to talk about your emotions, can in itself be hugely beneficial.

There are many women who have been helped by complementary therapies and some amazing anecdotal stories of success, but there are many others who have spent large sums of money on therapies that they end up regretting. If you can afford it and you enjoy it, then complementary therapies can certainly help you relax and improve your sense of well-being, but they may not be right for everyone.

'The doctor I saw was very alternative and he thought I was over-stressed and if he could get me to relax it would be all right. I knew something was wrong. I knew it wasn't just a question of taking selenium or whatever. There's nothing like rushing out from work sweating to get there, only to be told by some ageing hippy that you are very tense. I wish I'd had the courage to say, "No, that's not right for me."' *Julie, 40*

Chapter ten

Pregnancy Loss

Losing a baby can be a devastating experience, however early in the pregnancy it happens. It is believed that up to one in five pregnancies may end in miscarriage, and many eggs that have been fertilised don't implant successfully in the womb and continue to grow. Women may not always be aware that they are pregnant, let alone that they have miscarried, as it can happen when you would expect your period anyway and without any other symptoms.

The fact that so many women do miscarry at some point in their lives doesn't make it any easier to cope when you have lost a baby. Miscarriage is so common that we don't always appreciate how traumatic the emotional impact can be. As soon as women get pregnant, they inevitably begin to look forward to a future with their baby, and those hopes and dreams are lost when they miscarry.

The symptoms of miscarriage

The most common symptom of miscarriage is bleeding.

Sometimes this may begin as light bleeding, or spotting, or it may be immediate very heavy bleeding. It is important to remember that some bleeding in early pregnancy is surprisingly common. There may be light bleeding when the fertilised egg implants into the wall of the womb, known as implantation bleeding, or some bleeding around the time a period would have occurred. It is important to take any bleeding in early pregnancy seriously, but light bleeding doesn't necessarily mean that there is something wrong.

The other main symptom of miscarriage is abdominal pain, but again this is common in early pregnancy. Mild aches or cramps can be caused by stretching of the ligaments that hold the womb. If you have severe cramping pains, especially if they are accompanied by bleeding, it does suggest that there may be a problem, and you should see a doctor immediately. If you seek medical attention for a suspected miscarriage, doctors will normally do an ultrasound scan to see whether the pregnancy is still progressing normally, and may also want to do a pregnancy test to check the levels of pregnancy hormones.

Complete miscarriage

A complete miscarriage is the term used when a pregnancy ends and all the tissue in the womb has come away and been discharged. Most miscarriages happen in the first trimester, or first 12 weeks, of pregnancy. If you have a miscarriage after this, it is known as a late miscarriage, and the loss of a baby after 24 weeks of pregnancy is a stillbirth. This can happen for no apparent reason, although it is sometimes due to problems with the placenta or to an abnormality in the baby's development.

'The last miscarriage I had was at 22 weeks. I'd had a scan three days beforehand and everything was fine. I just started bleeding and having cramps at about two o'clock in the afternoon, and by eight o'clock at night it was all over and done with. It was very upsetting at the time, but you can't dwell on it.' *Ann, 43*

Incomplete miscarriage

Sometimes when a miscarriage occurs, parts of the placenta, sac or embryo may be left in the womb. Bleeding and pain will often continue after the miscarriage, and if this happens you should contact a doctor immediately. It may be necessary to have a minor operation to clear the womb if you have an incomplete miscarriage. This procedure is called an ERPC (evacuation of the retained products of conception), an unpleasantly blunt title. You will have a general anaesthetic and the cervix will be opened, or dilated, so that the inside of the womb can be scraped clear.

'At the 12-week scan, they said there was no heartbeat. They gave us all these leaflets, and a couple of days later I started to miscarry. Physically it wasn't too bad, but they said they'd scan me to see how it was going, and they said it was incomplete, so I had a pessary, like an abortion pill, to finish it off.' *Elaine, 39*

Missed miscarriage

A missed miscarriage, or delayed miscarriage, happens when there have been no outward signs that the pregnancy has ended, although the foetus has died or failed to develop.

'I went to an antenatal appointment. We'd gone through the whole antenatal routine as normal. As we were leaving I said I wouldn't mind just hearing the heartbeat. I felt absolutely fantastic and I was so sure I was pregnant. My clothes were getting too small. I went in there thinking, "Hear the heartbeat, then walk out of here," but there wasn't a heartbeat.' *Alison, 38*

Blighted ovum

A blighted ovum is a fertilised egg that has stopped developing. There is a pregnancy sac, but no foetus inside and this can be diagnosed by ultrasound scan. The medical term for this is an anembryonic pregnancy.

'I was at work when I started pouring blood. They called an ambulance and at the hospital they did a routine blood test when I gave a urine sample. They told me I was pregnant and I was having a miscarriage. I didn't actually know I was pregnant so it was extremely traumatic. I had a scan and I could see something on the screen. It was a blighted ovum, so just the sac was there but nothing in it.' *Emma, 33*

Hydatiform mole

This is a rare condition that occurs when placental tissue grows despite the fact that there is no foetus. Around one in every 1,200 pregnancies is affected by this condition. With a 'complete mole', the mother's egg has no nucleus so a foetus cannot develop, whereas a 'partial mole' occurs when an egg is fertilised by two sperm, which means it has too many chromosomes and cannot grow. With both types of molar pregnancy, large quantities of the pregnancy hormone are produced, so women are often very sick. If a molar pregnancy is diagnosed, it is usually removed under general anaesthetic.

Recurrent miscarriage

When a woman has several miscarriages in a row, usually three or more, this is known as a recurrent miscarriage. It happens to about one in every hundred women, and most go on to have healthy pregnancies afterwards. If you have recurrent miscarriages you may be referred for tests to try to find out whether there is one underlying cause, but it is often not possible to find a reason. Coping with one miscarriage can be very hard, but when it occurs again and again this may be really devastating. It can start to dominate your entire life, and women often find it helps if they feel they are getting the specialist help and counselling they need, and that their situation is being thoroughly investigated. There are a few clinics that specialise in recurrent miscarriage, but unfortunately not everyone can access this kind of support.

> 'I had three miscarriages. I was told it was old eggs and it was my age. Had I had a fourth one, they would have put it down for investigation. They weren't that bothered with me in particular because I'd already had six children. I think had I been trying for my first or second they might have been more understanding and tried to help a bit more. I just got told it was old age, old eggs.' *Ann, 43*

What causes a pregnancy to miscarry?

For the majority of women who miscarry, there will be no clear cause. Although we know some of the conditions that may lead to pregnancy loss, most women will not know which, if any, of these may be responsible. Early pregnancy loss is a common occurrence, and generally women are not offered any kind of investigation or follow-up unless they have experienced recurrent miscarriage. For many women not knowing why they lost their baby is not only frustrating, but also the cause of future anxiety.

> 'I had a lot of guilt about the miscarriage. I picked apart every second of every day that I was pregnant and thought about what I'd done. What had I done wrong? I said that to the doctor, and she said there's absolutely nothing. In some ways I would rather someone had said, "On this day you did this, and it was the cause." I can't do anything to prevent it happening again, and that is really scary.' *Clare, 34*

There are some problems that we know can lead to miscarriage. The most common cause is some kind of chromosome abnormality in the fertilised egg. This is believed to be responsible for up to half of all miscarriages, and is more common among older mothers. Women who have hormonal problems, polycystic ovary syndrome or endometriosis (see Chapter 6) also have a higher risk of miscarriage. Some women have antibodies that react against the body's own tissues or cause blood clots, or abnormalities of the immune system, which can cause miscarriage. Infections may also sometimes be to blame, such as uterine or vaginal infections or listeria.

An incompetent cervix can be a cause of miscarriage during the middle months of pregnancy. This rather odd term means that the cervix, which usually remains closed until labour, is not strong enough to hold the pregnancy. Eventually the cervix dilates under the pressure of the growing baby, and the pregnancy is lost. If this is suspected, it is possible to put a stitch in the cervix during early pregnancy, which holds it shut.

Although it is rare, some women have an unusually shaped womb where there may not be room for the baby to develop properly as it gets bigger. This may cause a pregnancy to end in miscarriage. Women who smoke are more likely to miscarry than non-smokers, and older women are at greater risk.

Testing and preventative treatment

You will usually be offered testing only if you have had

three or more miscarriages. This may seem very harsh, but the majority of women who have had one or two miscarriages do go on to have a perfectly healthy pregnancy afterwards. It is often only where there have been three or more miscarriages that there may be an underlying cause for the problem.

'They wouldn't normally investigate after two miscarriages, but I was lucky because I hit on a sympathetic doctor. They told me research has shown that the proximity of support actually has an effect on reducing the incidence of miscarriage. They were lovely people, it was very convenient and you could walk in and have a scan and see the heartbeat, or phone up and talk to someone at any time. It was fantastically reassuring.' *Emily, 53*

You may be offered chromosomal analysis of your blood and your partner's, and sometimes of the baby's too. Pregnancy loss due to chromosomal abnormality is common. In a very small percentage of couples, miscarriage may be caused by a chromosomal abnormality in one of the parents, which means that the embryo will have some genetic information missing, and some repeated. There is no preventative treatment for this kind of chromosomal problem.

Sometimes blood tests will show that there are high levels of antibodies in the mother's blood. If this is the case, a low dose of aspirin or heparin is sometimes prescribed.

Women may be offered blood tests to see whether they have polycystic ovary syndrome, as this is associated with miscarriage. If this is the case, hormone treatment may be offered, although research has not yet proved that this has any real benefit.

The womb may be examined using an X-ray, ultrasound or hysteroscopy (see Chapter 7) to make sure there are no abnormalities there, and doctors may also want to check that there are no weaknesses in the cervix if miscarriages have occurred after the first trimester. They may take a vaginal swab or do blood tests to rule out any infections.

There is much ongoing research into the causes of miscarriage, and some fertility clinics do now offer immu-nological treatments for women who have had recurrent miscarriages, particularly if tests show that they have raised levels of NK, or natural killer, cells which some doctors believe may play a role in causing miscarriage. These treatments are fairly new, can be costly and there is not yet any clear scientific evidence to prove that they are effective.

Miscarriage and future pregnancies

The majority of women who've had a miscarriage go on to have a perfectly healthy and successful pregnancy in the future. It is true that if you've had a miscarriage, you are slightly more at risk of it happening again, but even women who have had recurrent miscarriages usually go on to have successful pregnancies.

Ectopic pregnancy

An ectopic pregnancy occurs when a fertilised egg implants outside the womb, usually in the fallopian tube, although it can on rare occasions be found in the ovary or cervix. Normally once an egg has been fertilised by sperm in the tube, it continues slowly down to the womb where it implants about six days later. With an ectopic pregnancy, the fertilised egg gets stuck in the fallopian tube and starts to grow there. As it gets bigger, it stretches the tube walls and this is often very painful. There may also be vaginal bleeding.

An ectopic pregnancy often dies quickly, even before the period is due, and in these cases there is no risk. However, if it continues to grow and is not diagnosed, it can rupture the tube, causing severe pain and bleeding. A ruptured ectopic can be life-threatening.

About one in every hundred pregnancies is ectopic, but it isn't always clear what causes an egg to get stuck. In many cases, no reason is found. If the tube is damaged, blocked or very narrow, or if there are kinks or adhesions, this can trap the egg. Ectopic pregnancies can occur if there is a problem with the little hair-like cilia that line the tube and help the egg move.

Some women are more at risk of having an ectopic pregnancy than others. If you've had pelvic inflammatory disease or chlamydia, this can damage the tubes and increase the risk of an ectopic pregnancy. Endometriosis or abdominal surgery can lead to scarring in the tubes, which may be to blame. Your choice of contraceptive can also play a role here. Women who have IUDs (coils) sometimes have ectopic pregnancies, as an IUD only stops a fertilised egg implanting in the womb and cannot prevent implantation in the tube. The progesterone-only pill has also been linked to ectopic pregnancy.

How would you know if you had an ectopic pregnancy?

The main symptoms of an ectopic are pain and bleeding, along with a missed or late period. The pain is usually just on one side of the lower abdomen, although oddly this pain isn't always on the same side as the ectopic. There may also be shoulder pain, which is caused by internal bleeding, and bowel and bladder pain too. Usually a pregnancy test will be positive, but a home test doesn't always pick this up, and you may need proper blood tests to check. There may be other symptoms of pregnancy, such as tender breasts and sickness. If there is bleeding, it is not usually like a normal period. There may be spotting, or unusual dark watery blood (which is said to look like prune juice). Sometimes women feel very faint, dizzy or light-headed.

What should you do?

If you think you may have an ectopic pregnancy, you should seek medical help immediately. A pregnancy test will be carried out, and an ultrasound scan. If the pregnancy test is positive and the womb is empty, this can indicate an ectopic pregnancy. Sometimes a suspected ectopic pregnancy may be monitored for a day or two if the pain is not bad, but a laparoscopy is usually the next step to allow doctors to get a proper look at the tubes.

An ectopic pregnancy will never be able to grow or move into the womb. It is not viable, and so the most important thing is to remove it before it ruptures the fallopian tube. Sometimes, if it is diagnosed early, it may be possible to treat an ectopic pregnancy without taking out the fallopian tube, but it is often necessary to remove it entirely.

> 'I'd had symptoms that I thought were PMT. I'd had sore breasts and had been really tearful. Then I was just doubled over in pain, and I knew something was fundamentally wrong. I was rushed into hospital, and they said, "You're pregnant." I was adamant that I wasn't. Within a few hours I was in theatre and I lost one tube. It ruptured.' *Lisa, 32*

Ectopic pregnancy and your future fertility

If you've had an ectopic pregnancy, your chances of getting pregnant are reduced, and your chances of having a second ectopic are higher than average, particularly if it was caused by some kind of damage to the fallopian tubes. However, despite this, many women do go on to have successful natural pregnancies afterwards.

You will probably be advised to leave time for your body to recover from the ectopic pregnancy before trying for another baby, but it may take you a while to recover emotionally too. An ectopic pregnancy can be a hugely traumatic experience, and although some women feel they want to try to get pregnant again as soon as they can, others may need time to cope with their loss first.

Emotions and pregnancy loss

The emotional impact of miscarriage and ectopic pregnancy is often underestimated. As soon as women discover they are pregnant, they begin to feel involved with their unborn baby. Even when a miscarriage happens very early in the pregnancy, there is not just the physical loss but an emotional loss too. Many women go through a grieving process when they lose a baby, and part of their sadness is about the lost future they had glimpsed ahead. The raw emotion does fade with time, but there may be unexpected feelings of sadness on the baby's due date or the anniversary of the miscarriage for some years to come.

> 'It's recognising that there is something to grieve about, particularly with very early miscarriages. Some people have said it was ever so early, it wasn't really a baby, but the moment you see a positive test, you have it arriving. You've got it going to school, you've got it heading off to university.'
> *Corinne, 36*

Men and women often experience the loss differently, and it can be hard if you feel your partner is not responding in the way you'd expected or would like. Sometimes it can increase existing tensions, but other people find it brings them closer together as a couple. Men may feel they have to try to be strong in order to support their partners, and hide their own feelings.

Other people are often difficult to deal with. They may not seem to understand what you are going through, and often don't know how to react. They may have the best intentions, or be trying to cheer you up, but can end up upsetting you. Although friends and family are often very supportive initially, there is sometimes pressure to 'get back to normal' before you feel ready for this. Other people may not appreciate how long it can take to come to terms with what has happened.

'At work people did know I'd had a miscarriage because it had happened there. Some people just avoided me to begin with, wouldn't even look me in the eye ... I know they probably didn't know what to say, but I couldn't stand that.' *Emma, 33*

Many women experience depression after a miscarriage. You may lose confidence, feel very low and unable to cope. Others feel very guilty, as if the miscarriage is somehow their fault when in fact this is not the case at all. It may be helpful to get some support at this time, and counselling or a voluntary support organisation can prove invaluable.

Infertility and pregnancy loss

Pregnancy loss and infertility are both hard enough to cope with by themselves, but having to deal with a miscarriage or ectopic pregnancy when you know it may not be easy to get pregnant again can seem an impossible burden. Some women find it helpful to know that at least they have conceived, and believe this offers hope for the future, whereas others don't feel this way about it at all. Miscarriage rates are thought to be higher among women who have found it difficult to conceive, but this can be partly explained by the fact that they often know they are expecting at a very early stage, and that they may be older when they get pregnant.

'It was devastating, absolutely devastating, but at the same time I drew some comfort from the fact that I could get pregnant.' *Helena, 34*

'People kept saying to me, "I know how you feel, I've had a miscarriage," and I thought they had no idea. Everyone thinks that their miscarriage is the worst, but other people might get pregnant again. People said things like, "Oh well, at least you got pregnant," but you don't go into trying for a baby to have the pregnancy. That's not the aim, just to have a pregnancy. It's the baby you want.' *Elaine, 39*

Sometimes a miscarriage can be easier for friends and family to relate to than infertility, and couples who have a miscarriage after years of infertility are sometimes surprised by the sympathetic reaction of other people who may not have been very understanding about their fertility problems.

Whatever your situation or circumstances may be, losing a baby is always going to be a difficult experience, and it is perhaps recognising this and allowing yourself time to grieve that will help you to come to terms with what has happened and to look towards the future.

Chapter eleven

Emotions and infertility

Once we've made the decision that we want a child, not being able to achieve this for whatever reason can unleash a complex web of emotions. Reproducing is something we expect to be able to do, and when we start to have difficulties conceiving, this can raise all kinds of fundamental questions about ourselves, and our aims and objectives in life. Women often say that it is only when they emerge from the other side of the experience that they realise quite how much infertility has affected them.

Shock

The first emotion many women experience when they realise that they are not going to be able to get pregnant easily is shock. We grow up expecting that we will be able to have babies if, and when, we want to, and we just assume that we will be able to do it the straightforward way. There is a stereotypical image of the infertile woman as a sad, desperate and lonely person, and this is not how we want to see ourselves. Although we may judge female success in terms of career and money nowadays rather than proficiency at domestic duties, there is still a stigma attached to not being able to have children. Accepting that you are going to have to spend a lot of time and money at a fertility clinic is going to take a while to sink in, and feelings of shock may be followed by anger and frustration.

Isolation

When you are trying unsuccessfully to get pregnant, it can seem as if everyone else you know is either pregnant or has young children, and it is very isolating. You may suddenly notice how family-orientated our society is when you are longing for a child of your own. The world is full of babies and buggies, and it seems that you can't read a paper or magazine, switch on the television or go shopping without being confronted by constant reminders of what you can't achieve. The fact that you are surrounded by other couples who are also experiencing infertility, tends to be a lot less obvious, partly because we are often reluctant to talk about it.

Women sometimes feel that they start losing friends as a gulf in understanding and experience grows when you are trying to get pregnant, and one by one all your friends are slowly succumbing to the baby bug. Your friends' lives may be changing rapidly when they have young babies, their priorities are no longer the same, and they may not want to go out and socialise or do the things you used to enjoy together. What's worse, you may find you have little to talk to them about when their only topics of conversation are nappy rash, potty training or introducing solids. You may feel you are rapidly shedding friends, just when you need them most. It can take very little time for women who are trying unsuccessfully to conceive to feel cut off from friends and family, and from society at large.

'All my school friends now have children, and all our other friends all have babies. We don't know many people who haven't got kids now. You go out with your friends, and they're all talking about babies. You can't begrudge their happiness, but sometimes it gets to you when you're surrounded by it.' *Mikaela, 32*

Dealing with social situations

Those feelings of isolation can make certain social situations difficult. Christenings, birthday parties and family events may make you feel awkward, particularly if there are lots of children present. Meeting new people can suddenly become fraught with problems if you find yourself dreading the inevitable questions about whether you have children, and whether you'd like to have a family one day. Christmas, which we tend to think of as a time for children, can be hard, and is sometimes an unwelcome reminder that yet another year has passed and you still haven't achieved your goal.

'It's very awkward for my friends because they've all got children. I have tried to explain. I don't like going to children's birthday parties now because I feel like a spare part. I don't have a child, and I feel like I shouldn't be there.'
Monica, 41

Dealing with work

Work situations can be difficult too, particularly for those who have to deal with pregnant women, babies or young children on a daily basis. Women who grow up with a strong maternal instinct may veer towards careers that involve spending time with children, and when you find you can't have your own, your job can become much harder. It's not just working with children that can be difficult. Watching work colleagues get pregnant, go off on maternity leave and then come back again while you are still trying to conceive can be incredibly depressing. It is perfectly normal to feel jealous of other women's pregnancies, but dealing with these negative feelings is not easy.

'Every day I go to work in fear of an announcement about someone being pregnant. I really don't know how I am going to cope with it. I struggle seeing people in the street who are pregnant, I have to not even look at them. I feel like it's turning me into a really horrible person.' *Lisa, 32*

Feelings of shame and failure

Women who can't get pregnant often start to believe it is somehow their fault. Even though you know you haven't done anything to cause the problem, there may be a sense of shame, and a feeling that you have failed because you can't do something that comes so naturally to others. You may feel your status as a woman is undermined by your inability to conceive when friends and colleagues are getting pregnant and giving birth. These feelings are often accompanied by a sense of guilt for not being able to provide the child we know our partner and family are longing for.

'I felt I was so different to everyone else because all my work colleagues were going off and having babies and I couldn't do that. I felt I was such a failure, and I felt I wasn't a proper woman because I couldn't do what everyone else takes for granted. When I was in that depression I couldn't see anything other than failure, that we'd failed everything and let everyone down.' *Mary, 38*

Depression

It is clear that infertility is a major cause of emotional upset, and the vast majority of couples going through fertility treatment suffer some degree of depression and isolation. There may be a general sense of bleakness and gloom, which seems to pervade everything, and women often find that they feel sad and tearful. It can be hard to talk about the pain you are feeling, as other people simply

don't understand unless they have some personal experience of what you are going through.

Some women feel their infertility makes them into a
less likeable person. You may feel your entire personality
is changing, and that you have become jealous, angry and
brimming with negative emotions. Treatment may make
you feel low, and you may lose your sense of fun and
enjoyment of other areas of your life. It is easy to forget
the positive things in your life, as not being able to get
pregnant starts to dominate everything.

'When I wasn't getting pregnant, I used to wake up and the
first few seconds you think, "Oh, it's a sunny day," and then
all of a sudden the reality would hit you, "hang on, I am
still going through infertility." It was desperately painful and
really depressing when everyone around you was pregnant
and having babies.' *Claire, 44*

Coping with other people

Our friends, family and colleagues may not know how to
deal with our situation, and despite their best intentions,
can often end up saying the wrong thing. They may just
be trying to be helpful, or to cheer us up, but we have to
recognise that infertility does make us very sensitive, and
questions that might seem perfectly innocent to anyone
else can be really upsetting. Other people are not always
going to understand, however hard they try, and they may
find it hard to appreciate quite how devastating infertility
can be.

Losing confidence and control

The process of going through fertility tests and treatment can be demoralising, and normally forthright women sometimes find themselves becoming strangely meek when faced with a doctor who holds the power to help them achieve their dreams. The indignity of many of the tests and treatments is scarcely a confidence booster, and the lack of control over what is happening can make you feel helpless. Women often say they feel there is nothing they can do to influence the outcome of any treatment or to make things better for themselves. It can make you angry and frustrated, and this sense of powerlessness may be particularly hard for women who have been successful elsewhere in life.

> 'I hated not having what I wanted and not being in control. I don't think it helps if you are goal-orientated and competitive, used to working hard and achieving whatever you want to achieve. It was humbling for me to realise that we are in the lap of the gods, and that sometimes there's nothing you can do about things, no matter how much money or effort you put into them.' *Julie, 40*

The race against time

There is inevitably a lot of waiting involved in fertility treatment, not just during the two-week wait to find out whether you are pregnant or not, but also when you are waiting for appointments and referrals, for tests and results, and this sense that time is slipping away can be particularly hard if you are already worried about your age.

> 'I feel like I'm standing still while everyone else runs on past me. There are people I know who started trying after we did and are now having their second child.' *Corinne, 36*

Your relationship

The stress of infertility can take a toll on how you get on with your partner, and the emphasis on baby-making can affect your sexual relationship too. About a third of patients going through fertility treatment say it has a negative effect on their relationship. If one of you feels responsible for the fertility problem, it can cause guilt, and you may adopt different coping strategies. Some women say that they want to talk about the situation more than their partners and that infertility can be difficult for men to cope with. However, it is not just a matter of men and women dealing with things differently, and lesbian couples may experience strains on their relationships during fertility treatment too.

> 'When I first started trying to get pregnant, it had a huge effect on my relationship because it was very stressful. I always felt I was more obsessed about it, and I was getting more and more obsessive and my partner was getting more and more distanced from it all, and ultimately getting to the point where she felt she didn't want to have a child at all.' *Naomi, 39*

Research suggests that for every couple who find their infertility has a damaging effect on their relationship, there is another couple who find that going through such a stressful experience together strengthens their relationship.

'It did bring us closer all the time. I've seen people where they are driven apart and that's sad, but it just brought us closer because we were having to go through so much.'
Ann, 44

Grief

When fertility treatment is not successful, both partners can feel an overwhelming sense of hopelessness, and of grief. It may sound odd to experience grief for something you've never had, but we grow up with expectations about life, which may include having a family of our own. We may have imagined what our children might be like, and how we would want to bring them up, and there is a sense of grief when we realise we may have to let go of this dream. One of the most difficult things about infertility is that there is no knowing when it will end. We may feel there is no hope, nothing to look forward to, and no guarantee that there will ever be a conclusion to the situation.

Coping strategies

There are some strategies that can help you cope, even when everything feels completely bleak and hopeless. Just talking can be a real lifeline. Seeking out others who've been through similar experiences, informing yourself about all your options and taking time to rediscover some of the things you used to enjoy can all be beneficial

Counselling

Many couples start out feeling that they don't want, or need, to see a counsellor, and that they have a good network of friends they can talk to. This kind of support is invaluable, but there may be certain areas you can't broach with your friends, times when you don't feel they entirely understand, or when you simply feel that you must be starting to bore them with your problems. In these situations, talking things through with an independent counsellor may be the answer. Some couples are wary of seeing a counsellor because they feel it might suggest that they can't cope, but in fact it simply shows that you are doing your best to help yourself in a difficult situation.

'I see a counsellor at the IVF clinic. I've seen her two or three times and it is very helpful. It's not just confined to the IVF. We talked about problems with my job, and she said maybe that was somewhere I could actually take some control back, rather than feeling that my fertility was out of my hands and my job was out of my hands. She is very good.' *Corinne, 36*

Sharing the experience

Talking doesn't just help you deal with what is happening, it may also help other people going through the same experience. The more open you are about your infertility, the more likely it is that you will find others among your network of friends and colleagues who may be going through the same thing. Local support groups, national networks and online forums can all play a vital role, and are an invaluable source of information and advice.

Informing yourself

Learning more about fertility, about tests and treatments, is a vital step in regaining control over your life. Once you start to try to help yourself, and to inform yourself about your options, this will give you the sense of regaining some control over what is happening, and can help increase your confidence.

'One of the things IVF did for me was turn me into a massive investigator. I did loads of research myself because I like to be in control of my own destiny. I didn't find it as emotionally stressful or demanding as other people did because I really tried to stay in control as much as I could and not be shy of asking questions.' *Helena, 34*

Taking a break

You may feel you have stepped onto a conveyor belt you can't get off when you are going through fertility treatment, and sometimes couples find it useful to take some time out for a while to help put things back into perspective.

'You are on a roller coaster and because you are conscious of your age, you daren't take time out. The best thing I ever did was take two years off. We looked at adoption and I started doing things to help my confidence, which I had lost. I started running. I even went out and got drunk a few times. It made a difference to me, and a difference to my relationship with my husband.' *Alison, 38*

However hard it may seem at the time, there will be an end at some point. You may decide you can't face the thought of fertility treatment, you may feel you don't want to go through any more after having unsuccessful treatment, you may feel that you want to adopt or to try to learn to live without children – or you may be successful, either with medical help or naturally. Whatever happens, the experience of infertility may be dulled but will never entirely leave you. Women who get pregnant after spending years trying to conceive sometimes feel it has changed the way they experience pregnancy and motherhood. However, this change is not always negative. As hard as it can be to imagine when you are still going through fertility tests or treatments, you may feel at the end that you have gained some positive things from the pain you have suffered.

Chapter twelve

Other Ways to be a Mother

Being a mother doesn't have to involve using your own egg and your partner's sperm, it doesn't have to involve giving birth at all. Many women who cannot have children the traditional way discover that there are other routes to parenthood. Women may use eggs or sperm from a donor, or find another woman who is willing to carry their child in her womb, or they may decide to adopt. Although there is a wide variety of ways to become a mother, the job is pretty much the same no matter how you get there.

'If you are lucky enough to have a child, you just love that child. I don't ever think now that I wish my son had been from my eggs because it wouldn't have been him, and it feels so much like he was meant to be.' *Claire, 44*

Egg donation

Women who no longer produce their own eggs, whether due to age, an early menopause or to a medical condition, may choose to use donated eggs as a route to motherhood. Egg donation was first used successfully in the 1980s, and allows a woman who would otherwise be unable to have her own children to go through the whole experience of pregnancy, giving birth and breastfeeding her baby.

If you are thinking of using donated eggs, it may throw up some emotional and ethical issues you will need to grapple with. Counselling is essential, as you need to consider the consequences for you, your partner and your child. Some people start out by thinking that they wouldn't want to tell a child at all, but it is generally accepted that it is important for children to understand the truth about how they were conceived, and to appreciate how much they were wanted.

'Hopefully, they will understand. You are bringing them up to give them as much security and to cocoon them as much as possible. You give them your morality and values.'
Sophie, 43

One real problem with egg donation is the shortage of available donor eggs. In order to give eggs, women have to go through almost an entire IVF cycle themselves, taking drugs to stimulate the ovaries and then having the eggs collected. This is not something anyone would undertake lightly, and there is also the risk of hyperstimulation from the IVF drugs, which makes the task of recruiting egg donors a fairly difficult one. Some women find a friend or family member who is prepared to donate eggs, or they may advertise to try to find a donor.

'My friend inspired me. She decided to put up posters around the local town asking for somebody to donate for her, and I thought if she could do it, I could do it. I said I'd do some press, and I'd done a couple of interviews and put the clinic's name out. We got some people coming and donating as a result of our publicity, so they moved me up the waiting list.' *Debbie, 44*

If a woman is interested in becoming an egg donor, she will be screened to make sure she doesn't have any infectious diseases such as HIV or hepatitis. Women usually have to be under 35 to donate eggs, as older women's eggs have a greater risk of chromosomal abnormalities and are less likely to implant. Donors and recipients are matched as closely as possible to try to get similar colouring, racial background, height and weight.

Once the donor has been given the all-clear, she can start taking the drugs to stimulate her ovaries. Human eggs are fragile and do not survive the freezing and thawing process very well, so egg-donation cycles use fresh eggs. The recipient is also given drugs to synchronise her cycle with her donor's so that her body will be ready for the donated egg. The egg donor has her eggs collected, and they are fertilised with the recipient's partner's sperm. Then one or two can then be returned to the recipient's womb.

In some countries, such as the UK, Sweden and New Zealand, egg donors no longer have anonymity, which means that any children born from a donated egg will be able to find out about the woman who donated if they wish to at some point in the future. In some other places, egg donors are anonymous, and can never be identified.

The severe shortage of donated eggs has led to more and more women seeking treatment overseas. In countries where donors are paid and maintain their anonymity, there tend to be more donated eggs available. If you decide to be treated abroad, this may mean that your child's heritage will be very different from your own. They may wish to explore this in the future, and could feel thwarted by the fact that they may not be able to identify their genetic mother. There may also be many practical hurdles to overcome if you are having egg donation abroad. It's not just the travelling that can be awkward, but there can be problems with language and the fact that clinics in other countries may not be subject to the same rules and regulations. They may not offer any follow-up advice or support, and probably don't provide counselling. You may be asked to pay in advance or even to pay in cash, while some clinics offer a 'shared risk' policy where you hand over a large lump sum, part of which will be returned if you don't get pregnant after a set number of treatment cycles. You should always ensure you have done your research thoroughly before you opt for treatment abroad.

Where women are paid, there may be a wide variety of donors who may choose to donate primarily because they need the money. Altruistic donors, who don't get paid, are often women who have young families and who want to help another woman experience the happiness they have found from their children.

'I'd reached the stage in our own treatment where I was grateful for everything that was in place. I appreciated the fact that it had taken a lot for me to get pregnant, and I'd relied on a lot of people to get me there. If I'd found out I needed an egg donor, I'd have wanted somebody to be there for me, so it seemed to make sense that if I'd expected somebody to be there for me, I should do it. I did my first egg donation when my children were about eight months old, and then I did four more.' *Doriver, 41*

Some clinics offer egg-sharing schemes where younger women who need IVF are offered cut-price treatment if they agree to donate half their eggs to another woman who needs them. This can seem an attractive offer if you need fertility treatment and can't afford to pay for it, but counselling is really important if you are considering this.

'I looked into egg sharing, but there is no anonymity. You could have a young adult knocking on your door because someone else had been successful with your eggs. It could work for someone else and not for us. I would have done it because it helps other women who aren't producing eggs, and it's a reduced price for IVF, but it's just the thought of the years to come ...' *Gillian, 34*

Donor sperm

Couples with fertility problems have been using donor sperm since the 1930s, although the pioneering doctors who first used the technique met with considerable hostility from both the medical profession and the general public. Despite this, the use of donor sperm for male fertility problems became a very common form of treatment. The advent of ICSI (intra-cytoplasmic sperm injection, see Chapter 8) in the 1990s gave new hope to men who would have had to use donor sperm in the past. ICSI allows men with impaired fertility to use their own sperm, which are injected right into the eggs in order to fertilise them.

If you are using donated sperm, the insemination can usually be carried out in a normal cycle unless the woman has ovulation problems. ICSI, on the other hand, does involve going through the whole IVF experience with drugs and egg collection, and is more expensive. There are still some male factor fertility problems that cannot be solved by ICSI, and in these cases donor sperm may be the only way ahead. Donor sperm is also used by single women and lesbian couples.

Sperm donors are screened before they are allowed to donate, and their sperm is tested for infections such as HIV, before being kept frozen for six months. As with donor eggs, counselling is a vital part of the treatment process if you are using donated sperm, and any potential problems tend to arise when couples haven't had adequate counselling.

'We didn't have any counselling about using donor sperm. My husband didn't really want to do it until we decided that was the only way. The consultant sold it to us. He didn't suggest ICSI. He just decided donor sperm would be the best way to handle it and he said he could get donor sperm from a bank which had plenty in stock.' *Sonia, 34*

There are now shortages of donor sperm and some clinics have long waiting lists for those who will need to use it. Some women have always preferred to use known donors if they can find someone who is willing to donate, and this is an option that others may now want to consider. Using a known donor means a child can know who their biological father is, and may be able to build up a much closer relationship. Some donors want to be actively involved in the child's life, but many don't want any involvement. This is something you need to have discussed and agreed before going ahead. Women who don't have fertility problems sometimes carry out the insemination themselves at home if they are using known donors, but going through a clinic means the sperm will be screened and checked properly, and should maximise your chances of getting pregnant as your cycle will be monitored too.

Having an anonymous donor can cause difficulties for your child as they get older and you need to have considered how they will feel in the future about this if you have the option of using an anonymous donor, and what you will tell them. There are donor-conceived adults who have found it distressing not to be able to trace their genetic fathers, and although it doesn't inevitably cause problems, you do need to be aware of this.

'There are kids who will never be able to have any contact with their donor, and will never know anything about them.

I think that's quite hard for the kids. Even if my son never meets his donor, at least we know about him and I've got a picture of him, at least we have a bit of history.' *Ellie, 44*

Donor embryos

If there are serious problems with both sperm and eggs, some couples may both need to use donor gametes, or to use a donated embryo from another couple. There are fewer embryos donated than either eggs or sperm, and it can involve a long wait.

Surrogacy

For women who cannot carry a baby themselves, surrogacy is an option that may offer hope to those who have all but given up on the possibility of ever having a child of their own. A surrogate mother carries a baby for the couple, and hands it over to them after the birth. Surrogacy usually involves the use of the male partner's sperm, and may use an egg from the female partner, the surrogate herself or a donor.

In straight, or traditional, surrogacy, the surrogate uses her own eggs. She either inseminates herself with the male partner's sperm or goes to a clinic for insemination. This form of surrogacy is cheaper and may seem easier, but emotionally it can be more difficult for both the surrogate and the parents if she is making use of her own eggs.

With host surrogacy, the eggs of the female partner or donor eggs are fertilised in the laboratory using the male partner's sperm, and then returned to the surrogate's womb. This method is particularly helpful for women who are still producing their own eggs, but cannot carry a baby. It is more expensive and more invasive for the surrogate, but it may be less demanding emotionally for everyone concerned.

Whichever path is chosen, the surrogate will carry the baby and give birth, after which she will hand over the child to the intended parents who must then go through a legal process to become the official parents. Surrogate mothers do not get paid for what they do, but they are entitled to expenses. These can be substantial, and are not just the odd bill for folic acid supplements and maternity wear, but may cover for loss of earnings, travel, childcare, antenatal care, life insurance and even help around the house. During the nine months of pregnancy, these costs can mount considerably and surrogacy is not an option for couples with limited funds.

There have been cases in the past where a surrogate mother finds she cannot go through with the process she has started, and this is why it is absolutely vital that surrogacy arrangements are done through the proper channels. There are organisations that can help you find a surrogate mother, and who will work through the process with you. It is worth using any help of this kind you can access, as surrogacy is a complicated process and only those who have been through it themselves are really aware of all the potential pitfalls.

'You feel so disempowered because you are so desperate for a baby, and you're very open to being exploited. Our first experience was very negative in the end, and the surrogate terminated the relationship having said she would try with inseminations for up to a year. We had been looking at traditional surrogacy, but the way we'll be doing it this time is gestational surrogacy and I think I feel a lot happier with that.' *Claire, 44*

Adoption and fostering

'Once we started adoption, it wasn't about having a baby to substitute the baby we couldn't have, it was all about having a family and being able to do family things like going to the beach, going to the zoo. We've been able to do all those things, which has been amazing because there was a time when we never thought we'd be able to.' *Mary, 38*

Adoption is something many couples consider when fertility treatment hasn't worked, or they are told it is unlikely to succeed. It is a permanent legal way of finding a new family for children who cannot live with their birth parents. You take on responsibility for the child you have adopted, who becomes part of your family. Fostering, on the other hand, is a temporary arrangement where a child comes to live with you for a while but is likely to return to his or her family at some point.

The children who need adoptive families are often older children who may have brothers and sisters they want to stay with. They may have special needs or disabilities, and many have had difficult experiences in their early lives. This can make them quite challenging children to look after who may need a lot of time and attention.

Some couples prefer to try to adopt a child from overseas, where there may be more babies and younger children who need new families. If you do opt for this, you need to be aware that it can take a long time, and can be expensive. You will still need to go through the same assessments as if you were adopting at home, but there will be the additional complications of bringing a child from overseas. Many couples have adopted from overseas successfully, but you do need to have thought about the implications of taking a child away from their natural culture and heritage, and how you will deal with this as they get older.

The adoption process is fairly lengthy, as it is essential to ensure potential parents are right for children whose past experiences may have made them very vulnerable. There will be a detailed assessment carried out over some months, and once you have been approved to adopt you will then have to be matched with a child, which can take even longer.

'Adoption is just another roller coaster: off one and straight onto the next. There are long periods of waiting with big stresses, big highs and then the occasional crashing back down to earth with a bump.' *Nic, 33*

After going through years of traumatic fertility treatment, the decision to stop and go down another route to parenthood can be a relief. Most adoption agencies recommend that couples leave some time and space before they start on the adoption process if they have experienced fertility problems and treatment. It may take longer than you think to recover if you have spent some years going through treatment, or hoping to conceive, and it is important to give yourself a breathing space before leaping into adoption. Once you have decided to go down this path it can be hugely rewarding.

Chapter thirteen

Going it Alone

Many women find that their choices about when or whether to have a child are overshadowed by the fact that they haven't met the right partner. If you are aware of your biological clock ticking, and you want to have a baby before it is too late, this can start to dominate your life. Men have much more leeway and can afford to take time to make the decision to settle down, but, for some women, the fear that they may never meet the right person becomes overwhelming.

> 'I felt really desperate all the time; always thinking I wasn't going to meet someone in time. It's an awful lot of pressure. It used to consume me. I was going out on dates and meeting people, but never meeting somebody that I wanted to spend the rest of my life with.' *Susan, 34*

Changing expectations

We have much more freedom than our mothers or

grandmothers, and there is no longer the same pressure on couples to marry, settle down and start families. Women may not feel the need to have a male provider, and marriage is no longer an institution everyone has to buy into. However, most of us do still grow up believing that we will probably share our adult lives with someone else, but women often wonder how long they should spend waiting for Mr Right when they are getting older and less likely to conceive.

No one expects to find themselves in this situation, but when you are leading a busy life it can just seem to creep up on you. Women who have very successful careers often find that there is little time left for their personal lives, and although making the decision to have a child by yourself involves a huge shift in hopes, dreams and expectations, it may be a logical way forward for women who haven't found a partner but know they want children.

Not all women who opt to have children by themselves set out with the deliberate intention of doing this. Some women do have unplanned pregnancies, or get pregnant with a partner who finds he cannot commit once they are pregnant, and must then decide whether to go ahead with the pregnancy alone or to have a termination. For women who know they want to have a child, and who may be worried that they are approaching the end of their reproductive lives, this may feel like an opportunity to become a mother that they cannot miss.

The wrong relationship

Men don't have biological clocks, and although there is some evidence that they may become less fertile with age, they certainly don't have the same time pressures. Men in their thirties may feel that they would like a family one day, but have no great motivation to get on with it sooner rather than later. It can be difficult for a woman who knows she wants to be a mother, yet finds herself with a partner who is not ready for the responsibility.

'I was going out with somebody who was a commitment-phobe. He kept making it sound as if we were going to start trying for a baby and get married at any minute, but nothing ever happened. He spent the whole time insisting that he wanted to have children, and he was very convincing. Twice he said he'd try for a baby and then changed his mind and said he couldn't do it.' *Thea, 39*

Finding yourself with a partner who doesn't want a child when you are determined you do is not only a problem for heterosexual women. Lesbian relationships can be affected in just the same way.

'I'd been in a long-term relationship, and it split my relationship up. I was purely interested in getting pregnant. I think she was quite angry with me because she didn't want me to be making that choice. She thought I was choosing it over being with her, being in a relationship.' *Ellie, 44*

Thinking it through

Having a child by yourself is not a decision anyone takes lightly, and most women spend a great deal of time considering the consequences and implications of opting to become a lone parent before going ahead. There are some key areas that can cause problems, and you will want to have thought through them first.

Is it a selfish choice?

Many women thinking about having a child without a partner find themselves caught up in moral dilemmas about whether it would be selfish to bring a child into a lone-parent family deliberately. They may fear that they would be short-changing their child, and that being brought up without a father would be inherently emotionally or psychologically damaging.

The traditional two-parent family is still held up as an ideal (despite the fact that it is no longer the norm for many children), and a single mother bringing up a child by herself is often regarded as second best. In fact, the number of parents a child has is not going to be the most important factor for their future happiness, and a child would be more likely to flourish in a happy, stable one-parent family than an unhappy, unstable two-parent family. It is natural for anyone considering a child to think about these issues, and such concerns can be particularly acute for women who don't have large disposable incomes, and may fear that their child will suffer materially for being in a one-parent family.

'I did feel selfish because I thought I should be thinking of the child. He was going to be born into a life where he's only got me who doesn't earn a massive wage and doesn't have a great big house or anything. I think it probably comes from the way we were brought up. You don't have babies on your own, you just don't do it.' *Lynne, 36*

Can you afford it?

Although you don't have to be wealthy to choose to have a child by yourself, it is certainly much easier if you are financially stable. There are not just the costs of donor sperm treatment to consider, but also money to cover your maternity leave and the longer-term financial demands of having sole responsibility for a child. You do need to sit down and work out how you will support yourself during your maternity leave, and to ensure that your salary is sufficient to cover childcare costs and other expenses. It is worth trying to save some money if you possibly can, and aiming to pay off any outstanding credit-card debts. If you are planning to spend some time at home when your child is young, you have to be realistic about how much money you will need to live comfortably. Obviously, everyone has their own ideas as to what constitutes comfortable, and it is undoubtedly possible to live happily and frugally as a lone parent without large amounts of spare cash. However, it will be far easier if you are not constantly worried about how you are going to pay the bills.

Do you have a good support network?

A good support network of family and friends can really

make all the difference to the experience of having a child on your own. Women who have done it by themselves stress that it is important not to expect too much from your friends, who have their own lives to lead and may not always be able to give you all the help you would like, but you will need some support. Having people you know you can talk to, friends or family who can share some of the joys of motherhood with you along with the traumas, will make things much easier. New mothers often find that they feel lonely, whether they have partners or not, and making sure that you have people you can turn to is essential.

If you can talk to other women who have made the decision to have a child alone, you will find their insights and advice invaluable. They will not only be able to understand how you are feeling better than anyone else but will also be able to give the kind of practical advice you may not find elsewhere. There are networking groups for women who are lone parents, and for those who have had children after donor insemination, and they can offer helpful information as well as support.

'I would definitely say get your friends and your family involved. I've felt so supported. I think it really deepened a lot of friendships and I felt, when I finally did get pregnant and have a baby, as if we'd almost done it as a group. They were closer, much more like aunties and uncles than they would have been if I'd done it with a partner.' *Rachel, 42*

Accepting your decision
Although it is far from uncommon for children to be

brought up in lone-parent families, women who have actively made the decision to do this often feel that they face criticism and need to justify their choice. Having a child alone is not something you would necessarily have chosen to do, and women often resort to this because they are aware that time is running out, and fear they may miss out on the opportunity of having a child entirely if they keep waiting for the right partner to come along. The fact that this may not have been your first choice doesn't mean it is a bad choice, although you will have to come to terms with the idea that your future is probably not going to turn out the way you might have envisaged it.

'It was really hard accepting that I'd be having my first child at the very least on my own, that I won't know the father, it will be a stranger, I am not going to have a husband who loves me sharing this with me. Coming to terms with that took me quite a long time. Now I have accepted that I've got to do it this way I don't feel I am doing an immoral thing, just the best I can do in the circumstances.' *Thea, 39*

Telling other people

Telling friends and family that you are planning to have a child alone can be difficult. Whereas some people will be incredibly supportive of your decision, you have to accept that not everyone will understand. It may be particularly difficult to tell your parents, who may feel sad that their daughter is not going to share the experience with a partner, or worried about how she will cope. Other parents are just delighted that they will, after all, have the opportunity to be grandparents.

'My mother had made a few disparaging comments at various times about single parents and I was anxious about how she'd take the news. The doctor asked if I'd told her, and on my next visit to my parents, I broke the news. I couldn't believe the look of utter joy on her face. She had no grandchildren at the time, and had clearly always wanted a grandchild but had been very careful to hide her desire.' *Ruth, 45*

The practicalities

So how do you go about getting pregnant when you don't have a partner? The prospect may seem daunting, but can be surprisingly straightforward once you are sure it is the right way ahead for you.

First steps

The first step is probably to talk to your doctor. Some women do try to bypass this, but if you have your doctor on your side from the start it can be incredibly helpful not just while you are going through the whole process of donor insemination, which can take a while, but also during the pregnancy, birth and early motherhood. If your doctor is not going to be sympathetic, it is worth finding that out sooner rather than later and signing up with another who is.

'I did see one doctor who said you can't have children until you've got a husband, so you'd better go and find one of them first and forget about anything else. I am quite cross about that because it was one of the times I really needed someone to give me some encouragement to do this. The doctor I see now is absolutely brilliant about it and really supportive.'
Thea, 39

Most women in this situation do feel that they want to have their own biological child, to experience pregnancy and birth, but it is also possible for single women to adopt, and this may be an alternative route to motherhood for women who don't have partners. This is not necessarily a quicker, or easier, option, as you will have to go through some fairly rigorous examinations to make sure you would be suitable to become an adoptive mother, but it is something many single women have done successfully.

Finding a clinic and a donor
Until fairly recently, it could take time to find a clinic willing to treat single women, but this is changing and it is now much easier to get treatment as a single woman or in a lesbian partnership. Your doctor should be able to refer you to a clinic, and the main problem you could face is a waiting list for sperm, as many clinics are experiencing a shortage of donors. If you know someone who might be willing to donate for you, that can make it much quicker. Women choosing this option often used to do the whole thing at home themselves, but going through a clinic ensures that the sperm will be screened for infection, and checked to make sure it is healthy and viable. The clinic

will also make sure you are ovulating normally.

If you are using sperm from a sperm bank, you will have some choice about the donor. Women are usually advised to try to select someone who has their colouring and physical characteristics. Some women feel they want to be able to make very definite decisions about this, but others don't. Doctors normally suggest IUI (intrauterine insemination), where the sperm is inserted right through the cervix into the womb itself to maximise the chances of success, and this will involve a number of visits to the clinic to ensure that the insemination takes place at the right point in your cycle.

Counselling

Anyone who is considering donor insemination should be offered counselling, and your clinic should make sure that you have seen a counsellor before going ahead with any treatment. Counselling can help you work through any uncertainties you may have, and should cover the issues and implications you will need to have thought about. The counsellor will want to discuss your feelings and motives, and will try to ensure you have thought through the realities of bringing up a child by yourself. They should also talk through what you are going to tell the child about his or her father, and the way they were conceived. Most of these issues are likely to be things you have considered anyway, but it can still be useful to spend some time talking them through.

Your chances of success

Like any kind of fertility treatment, or indeed natural

conception, donor insemination doesn't always work the first time. It may take a few attempts, and this can be difficult if you are very aware of your age. Just as with natural conception, the chances of treatment working are reduced as you get older, and it is important to take this into consideration.

'The clinic were open and honest with me. I was 40 and they did say that the chances for women of my age were reduced, but there were no factors in my condition that led them to think I wasn't still capable of having a baby. It didn't work the first time, but I had already prepared myself for the fact that often these things don't work the first time, and the fact that it may never work. It did work the second time.' *Sally, 47*

Pregnancy as a lone parent

Once you are pregnant, the whole experience of carrying a baby, giving birth and then looking after your small child can be challenging in any circumstances. Coping with all this by yourself can be incredibly hard work, and it is often very lonely, even if you have established a good support network, and you should be prepared for this.

'I found in pregnancy the hardest thing was going to scans on my own, going to classes on my own. I felt very isolated. It's a very difficult experience on your own, in the middle of the night when you've had no sleep, there's no one there and you're stuck with a screaming baby and you haven't a clue. Even now I still find it quite difficult to deal with the isolation.' *Lynne, 36*

Motherhood as a lone parent

The reality is that having a child is never easy, and there may be added financial and emotional burdens if you are going through it alone. You will not only have to get through the tough times alone, but you may feel you don't have anyone to share the good times with either. On the other hand, there may be some positive aspects to being a lone parent, as you will be able to make all the parenting decisions, and to take sole responsibility for choosing how you bring up your child.

There may be little time for yourself, and this can make it harder to go out and meet new people and start new relationships. However, some women feel this actually gets easier when you have your child first. The desire for a child can put an intense pressure on fledgling relationships when you are trying to assess your partner as a potential parent from the first date, and although time and money commitments may make it harder, some women do meet a new partner after having a child.

Changing times

We tend to think that choosing to have a child alone is a modern-day choice, and it was certainly more unusual a generation ago, but donor sperm has been a possibility for single women for decades, if they could find a doctor willing to treat them.

'I did feel like a pioneer. I didn't know anyone else who had done it. It was very hard, but better than the alternative of asking chaps round to supper who otherwise you wouldn't really want to sleep with. I went to a clinic in London and they agreed to treat me. My godmother hit the roof that I was having an illegitimate child. It wasn't unheard of, but it was awkward. There was still that stigma then. Certainly things have changed in the last 20 years.' *Victoria, 63*

So, should I do it?

Making the decision to have a child alone may not be easy, but it is certainly no longer an unusual choice. What advice would women who have already gone it alone give to others who are considering making the same decision?

I can absolutely, hand-on-heart say, aren't I lucky this was possible? Otherwise I would have probably either had a bad marriage and been a desperate woman, or been a bitter, childless woman.' *Mary, 41*

'I'd say go for it. I know lots of people that have regretted waiting too long. I don't know anybody that's ever had a baby and then regretted it afterwards.' *Gwyneth, 43*

Chapter fourteen

Living Without Children

Whether you are actively child-free or involuntarily childless, you are part of a growing minority of women. Living without children is no longer unusual, partly because more women feel able to make an active choice not to have children, and partly because many others find the opportunity eludes them. Whether you see yourself as child-free or childless, it can still be difficult to feel comfortable in a world where the family tends to be seen as a cornerstone of society.

'The culture we live in is very child-orientated. Children are virtually treated like gods in some families, and everything revolves around them. If you don't have children and you're not a family, then you're somehow not part of the culture that is prevalent at the moment. There's a big child-free section and our voices are totally forgotten.' *Sara, 44*

Stopping fertility treatment

Making a decision to stop fertility treatment, and coming to terms with the fact that you don't think it is going to work for you, can be very difficult. Where you draw the line is dependent on how much you can take before you feel you've had enough. For some women, venturing just a short way down the treatment path is quite far enough, but others carry on pursuing their dream through decades of costly and invasive treatment which can soon become all-consuming. There may always be the temptation to think that you should give it just one more go, or to try a slightly different treatment or new clinic in the hope that it might be the key to having a child of your own.

It may be your doctor who effectively makes the decision to stop treatment. Clinics are judged on their success, and if they feel there is little chance of treatment working for you, they may advise you that you need to think about egg or sperm donation, or that you should think about stopping altogether. There will always be another doctor willing to take you on whatever your situation if you have the money to pay, but you should think carefully and be sure that a new clinic can offer an increased chance of success if you have already been advised to stop treatment.

Sometimes the deciding factor in stopping treatment is the fact that a couple have reached the end of their financial resources. Fertility treatment is expensive, and funding is often restricted. Couples may be reluctant to let money stand in the way of having a child, and end up taking out loans or scrimping and saving in order to fund their treatment, but there is a limit to how much you can reduce your daily spending, and to how much you can borrow. It can make life seem very miserable if you are spending large amounts of money you don't have on treatment that isn't working.

For some couples, the decision to stop treatment begins as a simple need to take some time out and give themselves some space. Fertility treatment is often over-whelming, and can quickly dominate your life. Once you have launched into the process, it takes on a momentum of its own, and it often needs considerable strength to decide that you are going to have a break. It is particularly hard for older women who are aware that their fertility is likely to be declining, and may feel as if every month away from treatment is a wasted opportunity. However, those who do manage to jump off the rollercoaster for a while usually find it very refreshing. Some find they feel more positive about returning to the clinic after some time out, whereas it may make others more certain that they cannot face any more treatment.

'We just needed some space. We started to give ourselves other goals. For the first time in three years, we started to make plans for the future that didn't involve children.' *Nicol, 33*

The decision to stop treatment can be relatively straight-forward if one or both partners have reached a point where they realise they cannot go on. You may feel, both emotionally and physically, as if you have reached the end of the line. It may come as a sudden realisation that you don't want to put yourself through any more, or you may move gradually towards this point. There will always be a sense of grief at the loss of a long-held dream, but there may also be an unexpected relief that you are finally free from the endless round of tests and treatment, and can get on with the rest of your life.

> 'I felt I had come to the end of my tether. I was starting to question why I was putting myself through this, why I was putting my husband through it. It wasn't how I wanted to live my life. It was starting to take over and it just became too much. It was a great relief in one way that I didn't have to put myself through this any more, but there was great sadness that it hadn't worked.' *Jane, 45*

When you are going through treatment, one of the most difficult things is the sense that your life is somehow on hold. You may put off making decisions, or plans for the future, because everything is dependent on whether you get pregnant. You may not apply for a new job, or go for a promotion, or move house, and your fertility problems may seem to dominate every area of your life. Once you decide to stop treatment, you may finally feel that you have got your life back again, and can start making plans for your future.

Coming to terms with childlessness

It will take time to come to terms with the idea of a future without children. If you've always expected to have a family, it involves a huge change in your hopes and expectations about your life. There may be times when you feel very angry about your situation, and the fact that fertility treatment didn't work for you. We all read in our newspapers about the latest advances in assisted conception, and about women in their sixties getting pregnant, so it is hardly surprising that there is a general assumption that treatment is a cure for infertility. There is far less attention to the relatively low success rates, and having your own biological child is often thought to be a simple matter of going to the right clinic or having the right treatment.

You may feel as if there is a gaping hole in your life at first, and it can seem that there will always be that sense of something missing. It is only when you gradually start to re-build your life again, and to re-adjust your perspective, which has probably been tightly focused on treatment, that this will start to ebb away. It is never going to be easy when other women announce their pregnancies, and you may always feel some envy, and a sense of loss. These are natural emotions in the circumstances, and if you can accept that, it will be much easier to cope with them.

You may find that your confidence is very low, especially if you have suffered the raised hopes and dashed emotions of fertility treatment for some years. You may have suffered depression and deep sadness, which has coloured the rest of your life. Many women say they feel they have let themselves and their families down when they cannot have children. You may know that your parents are sad not to have had the opportunity to be grandparents to your child, and that your siblings were longing for a niece or nephew. It can take time to build up your self-esteem, and to come to terms with the fact that you are not to blame for what has happened. Your life may not be the way you had expected or wanted it to be, but that doesn't mean it can't be rich and rewarding.

Living without children

'Every day in almost everything that you do, there is a reminder that it hasn't worked out, and that you are not part of normal society. You do feel separate all the time.'
Heather, 48

You may find that your life is very different from the lives of your friends and family, who may all have their own children. Although some of them will try to include you in their family life, others may assume that you would rather not be involved if they know your circumstances. Some women find that spending time with children is painful and upsetting, but others may enjoy having the opportunity to be around other people's children. It is important to make sure your friends and family know how you feel about this, as it will make things much easier for everyone concerned. Certain social events, and indeed certain times of the year, such as Christmas, can be particularly difficult. If you know you are going to find an occasion painful, you may want to avoid it altogether.

You will inevitably have to deal with other people's insensibilities at some point. Try to remember that they are not deliberately setting out to be hurtful, but they may not have the least understanding of how you feel.

Some women who have decided to come to terms with a life without children do find it hard to cope with the way our society seems to assume that women automatically become more empathetic and caring once they give birth, and that childless women are somehow harder and colder. You may well find yourself faced with these stereotypes at some point, and it is not always easy to ignore them.

Many women feel lonely and isolated when they are trying to come to terms with childlessness, and it can be difficult if you have built up close friendships with other women going through fertility treatment who go on to have children of their own. It may help to seek out people who are in the same situation, and you might want to join a support group or Internet forum for couples who don't have children. It is not easy to talk to strangers about your most intimate feelings, but it can help normalise an experience that may feel very far from usual in the world outside. Counselling can be beneficial too, as it will give you a chance to work through your emotions, and to work out some strategies to deal with them.

Many couples discover they start enjoying their lives again once they have stopped trying to conceive. You may be able to appreciate the good things in your life for the first time for many years. You no longer have to worry about your biological clock, or saving money to pay for more treatment, and you no longer need to wait to make decisions or to change your life. This may give you a new lease of life, a new energy and confidence to be able to go forward and achieve some of the other things you've always wanted. You have freedom, you have opportunities to make the kind of life-changing decisions others may not feel able to take and to discover what you find truly fulfilling. It is not an easy path, and there will be hard times along the way, but most couples do find that, with time, they manage to move on and to enjoy all the other things they have in their lives.

'I'd love to say I am completely fine with it, but there is always going to be an element of me, I think forever, that wishes I had children, but it's more in proportion now. There are so many things in our lives I am happy about that wouldn't have happened if we'd had children. It was a catalyst for our lives completely changing.' *Isla, 35*

Child-free by choice

Women who have made an active decision to be child-free sometimes feel that they are out on a limb too. Despite the fact that so many of us don't live in a traditional family setting with two parents and children, we still tend to see this as the norm. Those who step outside this can feel judged and misunderstood.

'There's a presumption that having children and a family is always a good thing, that it is automatically more important, more valuable. Parents and anything to do with children are deemed to be beyond criticism and that, more than anything, can isolate you. Just because I don't want children that doesn't mean I don't like people.' *Wendy, 37*

In fact, statistics suggest that more and more women

are coming to the conclusion that they don't want to have children. Some may have always felt certain about their choice from any early age, whereas others do feel a degree of ambivalence about motherhood. Women who know they aren't ready to have children, and are certain they don't have any maternal instincts, are often told that they will regret it later if they don't have a child.

Assumptions are often made about the lives and personalities of the child-free based purely on the fact that they don't have children. They may be expected to be rich, successful career women who are simply too busy for a family, but in fact, many women who make this choice are far from the stereotype. You do not need a wonderful career, or a great deal of money, to decide that you'd rather not have children.

'Most people who have kids assume that people who don't have children have a high-flying career or an expensive lifestyle, and think they can't afford children and don't have time for children, which all sounds a bit harsh. There are plenty of us who have normal mundane jobs and pretty normal mundane lives.' *Sara, 44*

In fact, it is in the workplace that the child-free often feel they suffer most discrimination. Parents may complain about the difficulties of achieving an adequate work–life balance, but employers are actively encouraged to offer family-friendly work environments, and there are often tax breaks and other financial incentives for those who choose to reproduce. Parents may get generous maternity and paternity leave, the opportunity for flexible working and preferential treatment over time off and holidays, which can leave the child-free feeling short-changed.

It can seem as if there are huge gaps in understanding between those who are child-free and happy with their choice, and those who have children and assume everyone else ought to want them too. Some parents find it hard to understand how anyone could deliberately choose to be child-free, and cannot always accept that it is possible to be truly happy without children. Women who have made an active decision not to have children tend to relish the freedom that their choice has given them. They can be impulsive, they can do what they want, when they want to do it. They are not tied down by responsibilities, and can enjoy spending time with their partners. They are perhaps the best illustration that it is perfectly possible to live a rich, fulfilled and exciting life without children.

Resources

Australia

Access – Australia's infertility network
www.access.org.au

Aussie Egg Donors
www.aussieeggdonors.com
Support and information for egg donors and recipients

Donor Conception Support Group of Australia
www.dcsg.org.au

Fertility Society of Australia
www.fsa.au.com
Information for professionals and patients

Polycystic Ovarian Syndrome Association of Australia
www.posaa.asn.au
Support network providing information and advice
about polycystic ovary syndrome

Ireland

....

National Infertility Support and Information Group

www.infertilityireland.ie

New Zealand

....

Fertility NZ

www.fertilitynz.org.nz

Information, support and advocacy for those affected by infertility

Inter Country Adoption New Zealand

www.icanz.gen.nz

Inter country adoption agency for New Zealanders

New Zealand Endometriosis Foundation

www.nzendo.co.nz

Support, information and education about endometriosis

Miscarriage Support Auckland Inc

www.miscarriagesupport.org.nz

Information and support for those affected by miscarriage

South Africa

....

South African Society of Obstetricians and Gynaecologists

www.sasog.co.za

Information about how to find a gynaecologist, and links to information about infertility

United Kingdom

ACeBabes
www.acebabes.co.uk
Support for couples who are expecting a child after fertility treatment, and those who have become parents after treatment

Aromatherapy Council
www.aromatherapycouncil.co.uk

Association of Reflexologists
www.aor.org.uk

British Acupuncture Council
www.acupuncture.org.uk

British Association for Adoption and Fostering
www.baaf.org.uk
Information about all aspects of adoption and fostering

CHANA
www.chana.org.uk
Support network for Jewish couples with fertility problems

COTS
www.surrogacy.org.uk

Advice, help and support for surrogates and intended parents

Daisy Network
www.daisynetwork.org.uk
Support network for women who have experienced a premature menopause

Donor Conception Network
www.dcnetwork.org
Self-help network offering support and advice about all aspects of donor conception

Endometriosis UK
www.endo.org.uk
Support and information for women with endometriosis

Fertility Friends
www.fertilityfriends.co.uk
Online support for couples with fertility problems

Endometriosis SHE trust
www.shetrust.org.uk
Support and information for women with endometriosis

General Hypnotherapy Register
www.general-hypnotherapy-register.com

Human Fertilisation and Embryology Authority
www.hfea.gov.uk
Regulates centres carrying out fertility treatment in

the UK, and gives information on clinics and their
success rates

Infertility Network UK
www.infertilitynetworkuk.com
Patient support network, offering advice and information

Institute for Complementary Medicine
www.i-c-m.org.uk

Kidding Aside
www.kiddingaside.net
The British Childfree Association

Mothers35plus
www.mothers35plus.co.uk
Information, support and advice for older mothers

National Gamete Donation Trust
www.ngdt.co.uk
Information and advice for those considering donating
eggs or sperm, and for those requiring treatment with
donor eggs or sperm

National Institute of Medical Herbalists
www.nimh.org.uk

Netmums
www.netmums.com
UK-wide network with local contacts and information
for parents

OASIS

www.adoptionoverseas.org
Information and support for those considering overseas adoption, and those who have already adopted from overseas

Pink Parents

www.pinkparents.org.uk
Support for lesbian and gay parents

Reiki Association

www.reikiassociation.org.uk

Single Parent Action Network

www.singleparents.org.uk

Society of Homeopaths

www.homeopathy.soh.org.uk

Stonewall

www.stonewall.org.uk
Promotes equality and justice for lesbians, gay men and bisexuals

Surrogacy UK

www.surrogacyuk.org
Advice, help and support for surrogates and intended parents

TAMBA

www.tamba.org.uk
Information and support for families with twins, triplets and more

The Ectopic Pregnancy Trust

www.ectopic.org

Information and support for those affected by ectopic pregnancy

The Miscarriage Association

www.miscarriageassociation.org.uk

Support organisation offering information and advice

The Multiple Births Foundation

www.multiplebirths.org.uk

Working with families and professionals to improve the care and support for multiple-birth families

The Register of Chinese Herbal Medicine

www.rchm.co.uk

UK Confederation of Hypnotherapy Organisations

www.ukcho.co.uk

Verity

www.verity-pcos.org.uk

Support network offering information and advice on polycystic ovary syndrome

US

American Fertility Association

www.theafa.org

Information and support for those affected by infertility

American Society for Reproductive Medicine
www.asrm.org
Organisation devoted to advancing knowledge about
infertility and reproductive medicine

Choosing Single Motherhood
www.choosingsinglemotherhood.com
Information on single motherhood

Fertile HOPE
www.fertilehope.org
Help for cancer patients facing infertility

Fertility Plus
www.fertilityplus.org
Information for patients by patients

International Federation of Fertility Societies
www.iffs-reproduction.org
International federation of fertility specialists

Resolve – The National Infertility Association
www.resolve.org

Single Mothers by Choice
mattes.home.pipeline.com
Support and advice for women who are considering having
a child alone, and those who have already had a child alone

The Fertility Network
www.thefertilitynetwork.com
Information about infertility

Glossary

Adhesions: Scar tissue. Adhesions are like sticky cobwebs which can glue organs together

Blastocyst: An embryo which has developed in the laboratory for about five days before it is replaced

Cervix: The entrance to the womb from the vagina

Chlamydia: A sexually transmitted disease which can cause fertility problems

Clomifene: A drug used to stimulate the ovaries

D&C (Dilatation and curettage): This is a common surgical procedure during which the cervix is opened and the inside of the womb is cleared

Egg donation: Eggs are donated by a fertile woman to help others who do not have viable eggs of their own

Egg sharing: Some clinics offer egg sharing schemes. A younger woman who needs IVF will donate some of her eggs to someone who does not have viable eggs of their own and in return will pay less for her own treatment

Embryo: A fertilised egg

Endometriosis: A condition where tissue similar to the womb lining, or endometrium, grows outside the womb

Endometrium: The lining of the womb which grows at the start of each menstrual cycle and is shed during the period

ERPC (Evacuation of the retained products of conception): This procedure is often carried out after a miscarriage. The patient is given a general anaesthetic whilst the cervix is opened and the womb is cleared.

Fallopian tubes: The tubes which lead from each ovary to the womb. Fertilisation normally occurs in the fallopian tubes when an egg is on the way from the ovary to the womb

Fibroid: A benign growth found in the womb

Follicle: The sac in which each egg develops

Follicle-stimulating Hormone (FSH): A hormone which stimulates the ovary to produce follicles

Gamete: A sperm or egg

Gonadotrophins: Drugs which are used to stimulate the ovaries

Hysterosalpingogram: X-ray of the fallopian tubes to check they are clear

ICSI (Intra-cytoplasmic sperm injection): A variation of IVF during which a sperm is injected right into an egg to try to fertilise it

IUI (Intrauterine insemination): A form of assisted conception where sperm is placed into the womb

IVF (Invitro fertilisation): Sperm and egg are mixed together in the laboratory to try to produce embryos which can then be put back into the womb

Laparoscopy: An examination of the reproductive organs using a tiny telescope which is inserted into the abdomen whilst the patient is anaethetised

Oestrogen: Hormone produced by the ovary

Ovarian hyperstimulation syndrome (OHSS): The ovaries can be over-stimulated when a woman is taking gonadotrophins during fertility treatment. If the condition becomes serious it is known as ovarian hyperstiumulation syndrome, and a woman will need close monitoring and treatment

Ovulation: The moment when an egg is released from a follicle in the ovary

Pituitary gland: A gland at the base of the brain which is responsible for hormone production

Polycystic ovary syndrome (PCOS): Women who have PCOS have small cysts on their ovaries, and hormonal imbalances which can lead to fertility problems

Progesterone: Hormone produced after ovulation which encourages the womb lining to grow

Index